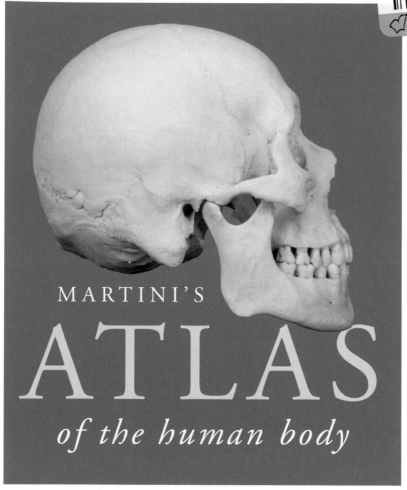

MARTINI'S ATLAS
of the human body

by

FREDERIC H. MARTINI, PH.D.

University of Hawaii at Manoa

with

WILLIAM C. OBER, M.D.
Art Coordinator and Illustrator

KATHLEEN WELCH, M.D.
Clinical Consultant

CLAIRE E. OBER, R.N.
Illustrator

RALPH T. HUTCHINGS
Biomedical Photographer

PEARSON

Boston   Columbus   Indianapolis   New York   San Francisco   Upper Saddle River
Amsterdam   Cape Town   Dubai   London   Madrid   Milan   Munich   Paris   Montréal   Toronto
Delhi   Mexico City   São Paulo   Sydney   Hong Kong   Seoul   Singapore   Taipei   Tokyo

Executive Editor: Leslie Berriman
Associate Project Editor: Lisa Damerel
Assistant Editor: Cady Owens
Editorial Assistant: Sharon Kim
Director of Development: Barbara Yien
Managing Editor: Mike Early
Project Manager: Caroline Ayres

Production Management and Composition: S4Carlisle
    Publishing Services, Inc.
Interior Designer: S4Carlisle Publishing Services, Inc.
Cover Designer: Derek Bacchus
Photo Researcher: Maureen Spuhler
Senior Procurement Specialist: Stacey Weinberger
Senior Marketing Manager: Allison Rona

Cover Photo Credit: Pearson Education.

Photo Credits: Author photos (p. iii, left to right): PK Martini, William C. Ober and Claire E. Ober, PK Martini, William C. Ober and Claire E. Ober, Ralph T. Hutchings. 1a, b, 2b, 3c, d, 4a–c, 5a–f, 7a–d, 8a–d, 9a–c, 10, 11a, c, 12a, 14a–d, 15a, c, 16a–c, 18a–c, 19, 20a, 21a–e, 22a–c, 23a, b, 24a, d, 25, 26a, b, 27d, 28, 29a–c, 31, 32, 33b, d, 34a–d, 35a, b, e, f, 36a, b, 37b, 38a, d–f, 39c, 40b, 41a, 42a, b, 43a–d, 44a, b, 45b, d, 46a, b, 49b–e, 51a–d, 52, 53a, b, 54a–c, 55a, b, 57a, b, 60a, b, 61a–c, 63, 64, 65, 66, 68b, c, 70a, b, 72a, 73a, b, 74, 75a–d, 76b, 77, 79a, b, 80a, b, 81b, 82b, 83a, b, 84a, b, 85b, 86a, b, 87b, 88b, 89, 90a, b Ralph T. Hutchings. 2a, 13f, 23c, 35c, 35g, 38b, 78a Patrick M. Timmons/Michael J. Timmons. 3a, 17, 27a–c, 30, 33c, 36, 37a, 39a, d, 40a, 68a, 69a, 76a, 81a, 82a, 87a Mentor Networks, Inc. 6 Image provided by The Digital Cadaver™ Project, courtesy of Visible Productions, Inc. 11b, 12b–d, 13b–e, 20b, 56a–c, 58a–c, 72b, 78b–g, 86c, 87c Frederic H. Martini, Inc. 13a Pat Lynch/Photo Researchers, Inc. 13g, 24c, 33a, 39b, 54d, 59, 69b, 85a Custom Medical Stock Photo, Inc. 15b, 53c Brendon G. Tillman/Naval Medical Center San Diego. 35d Peter Nguyen/iStock/Thinkstock/Getty Images. 38c, 47a–d, 49a, 62a, b Pearson Education, PH College. 42c Innerspace Imaging/Science Source. 42d, 67 CNRI/Science Photo Library/Photo Researchers, Inc. 44c C. Carl Jaffe, Diagnostic Imaging Branch Cancer Imaging Program, Division of Cancer Treatment and Diagnosis, National Cancer Institute. 45a, 71a Living Art Enterprises, LLC/Science Source. 45c Science Photo Library/Photo Researchers, Inc. 48b Marconi Medical Systems, Inc. 48c, 50a, 71b, 78i www.NetAnatomy.com. 50b Biophoto Associates/Science Source. 50c, 53d Christopher J. Bodin, M.D., Tulane University Medical Center. 53e P. M. Motta, A. Caggiati, G. Macchiarelli/Science Photo Library/Photo Researchers, Inc. 56d–f, 58d–f Visible Human Project/National Institutes of Health, National Library of Medicine. 78h Michael L. Richardson; University of Washington School of Medicine, Dept. of Radiology: www.rad.washington.edu.

Library of Congress Cataloging-in-Publication Data

Martini, Frederic, author.
    Martini's atlas of the human body/by Frederic H. Martini; with William C. Ober, Kathleen Welch, Claire E. Ober, Ralph T. Hutchings
        p. ; cm.
    Atlas of the human body
    ISBN-13: 978-0-321-94072-8
    ISBN-10: 0-321-94072-5
I. Ober, William C.   II. Welch, Kathleen   III. Ober, Claire E.
    IV. Title: Atlas of the human body.
    [DNLM: 1. Anatomy—Atlases.   2. Physiology—Atlases. QS 17]
    QM25
    612.0022'2—dc23   2014000640

 3 4 5 6 7 8 9 10-DOM-18 17 16 15 14

www.pearsonhighered.com

ISBN 10: 0-321-94072-5
ISBN 13: 978-0-321-94072-8

Frederic (Ric) H. Martini, Ph.D.
Author

Dr. Martini received his Ph.D. from Cornell University in comparative and functional anatomy for work on the pathophysiology of stress. In addition to professional publications that include journal articles and contributed chapters, technical reports, and magazine articles, he is the lead author of ten undergraduate texts on anatomy and physiology or anatomy. Dr. Martini is currently affiliated with the University of Hawaii at Manoa and has a long-standing bond with the Shoals Marine Laboratory, a joint venture between Cornell University and the University of New Hampshire. He has been active in the Human Anatomy and Physiology Society (HAPS) for over 20 years and was a member of the committee that established the course curriculum guidelines for A&P. He is now a President Emeritus of HAPS after serving as President-Elect, President, and Past President over 2005–2007. Dr. Martini is also a member of the American Physiological Society, the American Association of Anatomists, the Society for Integrative and Comparative Biology, the Australia/New Zealand Association of Clinical Anatomists, the Hawaii Academy of Science, the American Association for the Advancement of Science, and the International Society of Vertebrate Morphologists.

Kathleen Welch, M.D.
Clincal Consultant

Dr. Welch received her B.A. from the University of Wisconsin–Madison, her M.D. from the University of Washington in Seattle, and did her residency in Family Practice at the University of North Carolina in Chapel Hill. Participating in the Seattle WWAMI rural medical education program, she studied in Fairbanks, Anchorage, and Juneau, Alaska, with time in Boise, Idaho, and Anacortes, Washington, as well. For two years, she served as Director of Maternal and Child Health at the LBJ Tropical Medical Center in American Samoa and subsequently was a member of the Department of Family Practice at the Kaiser Permanente Clinic in Lahaina, Hawaii, and on the staff at Maui Memorial Hospital. She has been in private practice since 1987 and is licensed to practice in Hawaii and Washington State. Dr. Welch is a Fellow of the American Academy of Family Practice and a member of the Maui County Medical Society and the Human Anatomy and Physiology Society (HAPS). With Dr. Martini, she has coauthored both a textbook on anatomy and physiology and the *A&P Applications Manual*. She and Dr. Martini were married in 1979, and they have one son.

William C. Ober, M.D.
Art Coordinator and Illustrator

Dr. Ober received his undergraduate degree from Washington and Lee University and his M.D. from the University of Virginia. He also studied in the Department of Art as Applied to Medicine at Johns Hopkins University. After graduation, Dr. Ober completed a residency in Family Practice and later was on the faculty at the University of Virginia in the Department of Family Medicine and in the Department of Sports Medicine. He also served as Chief of Medicine of Martha Jefferson Hospital in Charlottesville, VA. He is currently a Visiting Professor of Biology at Washington and Lee University, where he has taught several courses and led student trips to the Galápagos Islands. He was on the Core Faculty at Shoals Marine Laboratory for 24 years, where he taught Biological Illustration every summer. Dr. Ober has collaborated with Dr. Martini on all of his textbooks in every edition.

Claire E. Ober, R.N.
Illustrator

Claire E. Ober, R.N., B.A., practiced family, pediatric, and obstetric nursing before turning to medical illustration as a full-time career. She returned to school at Mary Baldwin College, where she received her degree with distinction in studio art. Following a five-year apprenticeship, she has worked as Dr. Ober's partner in Medical & Scientific Illustration since 1986. She was on the Core Faculty at Shoals Marine Laboratory and co-taught the Biological Illustration course with Dr. Ober for 24 years. The textbooks illustrated by Medical & Scientific Illustration have won numerous design and illustration awards.

Ralph T. Hutchings
Biomedical Photographer

Mr. Hutchings was associated with Royal College of Surgeons for 20 years. An engineer by training, he has focused for years on photographing the structure of the human body. The result has been a series of color atlases, including the *Color Atlas of Human Anatomy,* the *Color Atlas of Surface Anatomy,* and *The Human Skeleton* (all published by Mosby-Yearbook Publishing). For his anatomical portrayal of the human body, the International Photographers Association has chosen Mr. Hutchings as the best photographer of humans in the twentieth century. He lives in North London, where he tries to balance the demands of his photographic assignments with his hobbies of early motor cars and airplanes.

For students in an introductory level anatomy and physiology course, an interpretive anatomical illustration is often the best way to introduce important information without distracting clutter. However, for true understanding, it is important to relate that interpretive view to "real world" anatomy, which is usually much more complex. For example, it is easier to learn the distribution of the major arteries in images that show only arterial and skeletal structures, and yet the concepts learned in that way can be hard to apply and interpret when dealing with a cadaver dissection or a hospital emergency. You might initially think that the best solution would be for a textbook to present illustrations in pairs—an interpretive drawing in conjunction with a matching "real" view such as a cadaver photo or medical scan. In fact, that is how many figures in my textbooks are organized. But to do that globally, for all structures and all systems, would be impractical and unwieldy. First of all, the same photographs would have to appear multiple times—the same image of the dissection of the forearm, for instance, would be paired with illustrations dealing with the bones, muscles, nerves, arteries, veins, and lymphatics of the forearm. Even if this redundancy were tolerable, the textbook would double in length unless the illustrations were reduced in size by half—an unacceptable option because larger images enhance understanding.

This *Atlas* solves that dilemma and makes it easy to relate clear diagrammatic illustrations in the textbook to the real world of dissection images and medical scans. It is designed to supplement the anatomical illustrations in Martini/Nath/Bartholomew *Fundamentals of Anatomy & Physiology,* Tenth Edition. Figure captions in that textbook indicate the related numbered plates in this *Atlas.* Together, that textbook and this *Atlas* provide a comprehensive and highly-visual orientation to the anatomy of the human body. Because it contains such a comprehensive series of images, this *Atlas* is also a useful companion for my other textbooks, including: Martini/Ober/Nath/Bartholomew/Petti *Visual Anatomy & Physiology;* Martini/Timmons/Tallitsch *Human Anatomy;* Martini/Bartholomew *Essentials of Anatomy & Physiology;* Martini/Ober/Bartholomew/Nath *Visual Essentials of Anatomy & Physiology;* and Martini/Nath *Anatomy & Physiology*—all available from Pearson Education.

The images in this *Atlas* are regionally organized. In key areas of the body, diagnostic medical images are paired with cadaver views. This will help students take an additional step—first from the diagrammatic illustration (in the textbook) to a cadaver dissection in a laboratory setting, and then from that inert cadaver to a medical image of a living person. The Contents also includes three quick reference guides for bones, clinical/diagnostic scans, and soft tissue anatomy.

This *Atlas* also contains a visual summary of human embryological development. The timing and depth of coverage of this topic vary widely across classrooms; some instructors cover the embryological development of individual body systems as they discuss each system, whereas others use the topic to wrap up the end of the course, or address the topic briefly only at the beginning and end of the course. There is general agreement, however, that understanding the key events in anatomical development requires an ability to visualize events happening in three-dimensional space. So in the Embryology Summaries section of the *Atlas,* we have created a visual presentation that pairs each written description with interpretive art. Students and instructors can refer to the sub-sections in the Embryology Summaries section, identified by topic and body system, as needed as your course proceeds.

In the preparation of this *Atlas* I have been very fortunate to work with Ralph Hutchings, considered by many to be the world's preeminent anatomical photographer, and Dr. William Ober and Mrs. Claire Ober, superb and creative medical illustrators who worked with me on the complexities of labeling the plates and helped create the Embryology Summaries. I would also like to thank the instructors who contacted me over the last three years with suggestions for the reorganization and improvement of this *Atlas.*

I hope you find this *Atlas* useful. If you have comments or suggestions for improvement, please contact me at the address below.

Frederic H. Martini
martini@pearson.com

CONTENTS

QUICK REFERENCE GUIDE TO BONES

QUICK REFERENCE GUIDE TO CLINICAL/DIAGNOSTIC SCANS

Gross Anatomy Plates

Skull

Clavicle

Scapula

Humerus

Ribs

Vertebrae

Radius

Ulna

Os coxae

Carpal bones

Metacarpal bones

Phalanges

Femur

Patella

Tibia

Fibula

Tarsal bones

Metatarsal bones

Phalanges

Skull

Clavicle

Scapula

Humerus

Ribs

Vertebrae

Radius

Ulna

Sacrum

Coccyx

Femur

Tibia

Fibula

Calcaneus

PLATE **1a** THE SKELETON, ANTERIOR VIEW

PLATE **1b** THE SKELETON, POSTERIOR VIEW

Occipital
bone

Spinal cord
emerging
from
foramen
magnum

Cervical
plexus
(C_1– C_5)

Cervical
spinal
nerves
(C_1 to C_8)

Brachial
plexus
(C_5– T_1)

Thoracic
spinal
nerves
(T_1 to T_{12})

Lumbar
spinal
nerves
(L_1 to L_5)

Lumbar
plexus
(T_{12}– L_4)

Sciatic
nerve

Sacral
spinal
nerves
(S_1 to S_5)
emerging
from
sacral
foramina

Sacral plexus
(L_4– S_4)

Coccygeal nerves (Co_1)

PLATE 2a THE VERTEBRAL COLUMN AND SPINAL NERVES

Cervical
vertebrae

Thoracic
vertebrae

Lumbar
vertebrae

Sacral
vertebrae

Coccygeal
vertebrae

PLATE 2b THE VERTEBRAL COLUMN, LATERAL VIEW

PLATE **3a** SURFACE ANATOMY OF THE
HEAD AND NECK, ANTERIOR VIEW

Supraorbital margin

Auricle (external ear)

Zygomatic bone

Body of mandible

Mental protuberance

Thyroid cartilage

Trapezius muscle

Cricoid cartilage

Clavicle

Sternocleidomastoid muscle (clavicular head)

Suprasternal notch

Sternum (manubrium)

Sternocleidomastoid muscle (sternal head)

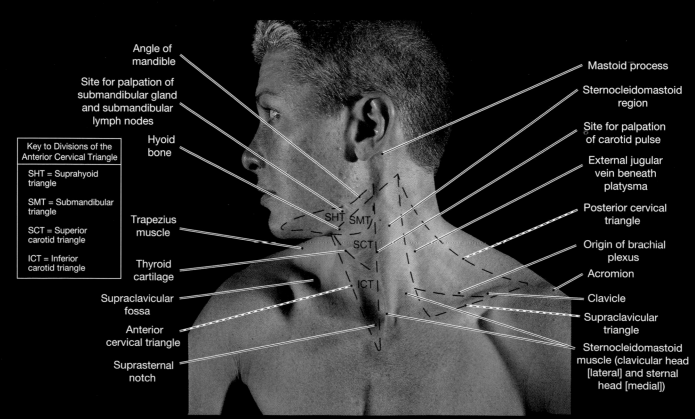

Angle of mandible

Mastoid process

Site for palpation of submandibular gland and submandibular lymph nodes

Sternocleidomastoid region

Site for palpation of carotid pulse

Hyoid bone

External jugular vein beneath platysma

Key to Divisions of the Anterior Cervical Triangle

SHT = Suprahyoid triangle

SMT = Submandibular triangle

SCT = Superior carotid triangle

ICT = Inferior carotid triangle

Trapezius muscle

Posterior cervical triangle

Origin of brachial plexus

Thyroid cartilage

Acromion

Supraclavicular fossa

Clavicle

Anterior cervical triangle

Supraclavicular triangle

Suprasternal notch

Sternocleidomastoid muscle (clavicular head [lateral] and sternal head [medial])

SHT   SMT
SCT
ICT

PLATE **3b** THE CERVICAL TRIANGLES

Epicranial aponeurosis

Frontalis muscle

Corrugator supercilii muscle

Temporoparietalis muscle

Orbicularis oculi muscle

Procerus muscle

Levator labii
superioris muscle

Nasalis muscle

Zygomaticus minor muscle

Parotid
salivary gland

Levator anguli oris muscle

Zygomaticus major muscle

Masseter muscle

Orbicularis oris
muscle

Buccinator muscle

Facial vein

Depressor labii
inferioris muscle

Facial artery

Mandible

Depressor anguli
oris muscle

Sternocleidomastoid
muscle

PLATE 3C SUPERFICIAL DISSECTION OF THE FACE, ANTEROLATERAL VIEW

PLATE 3d SUPERFICIAL DISSECTION OF THE FACE, LATERAL VIEW

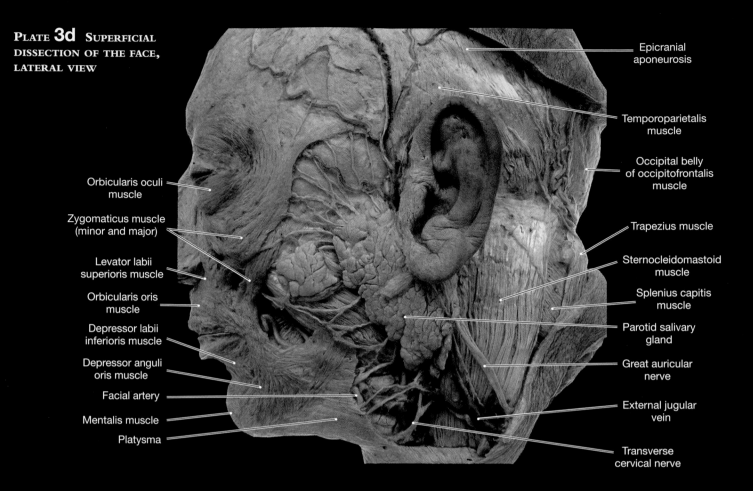

Orbicularis oculi muscle

Zygomaticus muscle (minor and major)

Levator labii superioris muscle

Orbicularis oris muscle

Depressor labii inferioris muscle

Depressor anguli oris muscle

Facial artery

Mentalis muscle

Platysma

Epicranial aponeurosis

Temporoparietalis muscle

Occipital belly of occipitofrontalis muscle

Trapezius muscle

Sternocleidomastoid muscle

Splenius capitis muscle

Parotid salivary gland

Great auricular nerve

External jugular vein

Transverse cervical nerve

PLATE 4a PAINTED SKULL, LATERAL VIEW

Frontal bone

Sphenoid

Ethmoid

Lacrimal bone

Nasal bone

Zygomatic bone

Maxillary bone

Mandible

Parietal bone

Occipital bone

Temporal bone

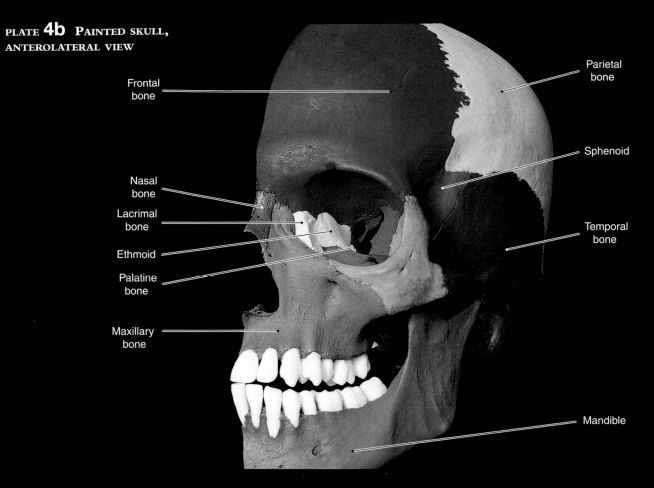

Frontal
bone

Parietal
bone

Sphenoid

Nasal
bone

Lacrimal
bone

Ethmoid

Palatine
bone

Temporal
bone

Maxillary
bone

Mandible

Frontal
bone

Frontal
sinus

Crista
galli
(ethmoid)

Parietal
bone

Superior nasal
concha
(ethmoid)

Middle nasal
concha
(ethmoid)

Sphenoid

Inferior nasal
concha

Maxillary
bone

Palatine
bone

Occipital
bone

Temporal
bone

Foramen
magnum

Mandible

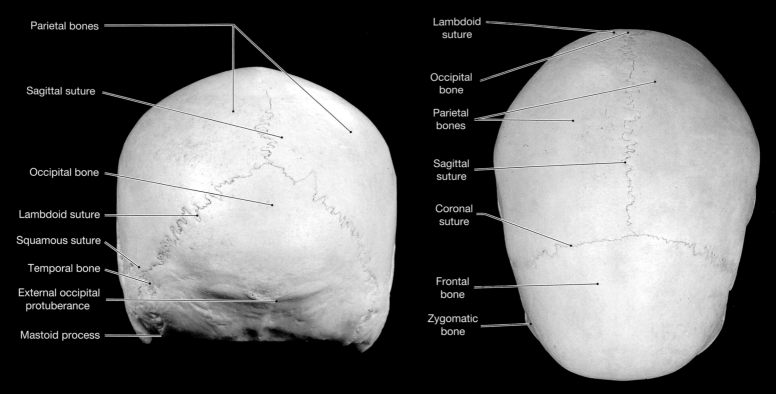

Parietal bones

Sagittal suture

Occipital bone

Lambdoid suture

Squamous suture

Temporal bone

External occipital
protuberance

Mastoid process

Lambdoid
suture

Occipital
bone

Parietal
bones

Sagittal
suture

Coronal
suture

Frontal
bone

Zygomatic
bone

PLATE 5a ADULT SKULL, POSTERIOR VIEW

PLATE 5b ADULT SKULL, SUPERIOR VIEW

Parietal bone

Superior temporal line

Squamous suture

Squamous part of
temporal bone

Zygomatic process of
temporal bone

Lambdoid suture

Occipital bone

External occipital
protuberance

Mastoid process

External acoustic meatus

Styloid process

Coronal suture

Frontal bone

Sphenoid

Supraorbital foramen

Ethmoid

Frontonasal suture

Nasal bone

Nasolacrimal groove
of lacrimal bone

Infraorbital foramen

Zygomatic bone

Maxillary bone

Mental foramen

Mental protuberance

Temporal process
of zygomatic bone

PLATE 5c ADULT SKULL, LATERAL VIEW

Greater palatine foramen

Lesser palatine foramen

Zygomatic bone

Sphenoid

Mandibular fossa

Jugular foramen

Styloid process

Stylomastoid foramen

Temporal bone

Hypoglossal canal

Occipitomastoid suture

Condyloid fossa

Lambdoid suture

Superior nuchal line

External occipital
protuberance

Incisive fossa

Maxillary bone

Palatine bone

Medial and lateral
pterygoid processes

Vomer

Zygomatic arch

Foramen ovale

Foramen spinosum

Foramen lacerum

Carotid canal

Mastoid process

Occipital condyle

Foramen magnum

Occipital bone

PLATE 5d ADULT SKULL, INFERIOR VIEW (MANDIBLE REMOVED)

PLATE 5e ADULT SKULL, ANTERIOR VIEW

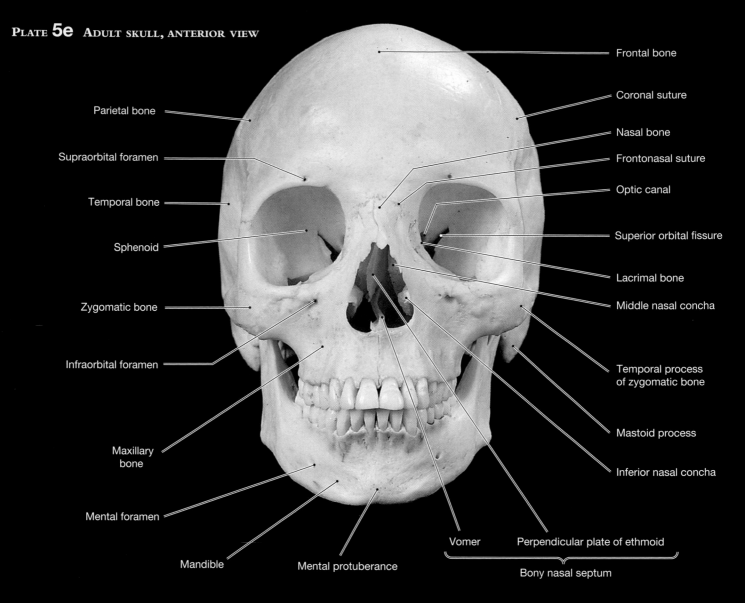

Frontal bone

Coronal suture

Nasal bone

Frontonasal suture

Optic canal

Superior orbital fissure

Lacrimal bone

Middle nasal concha

Temporal process
of zygomatic bone

Mastoid process

Inferior nasal concha

Parietal bone

Supraorbital foramen

Temporal bone

Sphenoid

Zygomatic bone

Infraorbital foramen

Maxillary
bone

Mental foramen

Mandible

Mental protuberance

Vomer   Perpendicular plate of ethmoid

Bony nasal septum

Frontal bone   Supraorbital notch

Sphenoid

Optic canal

Superior orbital
fissure

Infraorbital
groove

Inferior orbital
fissure

Zygomatic
bone

Maxillary
bone

Infraorbital
foramen

Ethmoid

Nasal
bone

Nasolacrimal
canal of
lacrimal bone
and maxillary
bone

PLATE 5f THE ORBITAL COMPLEX

Parietal bones

Frontal bone

Nasal bones

Zygomatic bone

Ethmoid

Maxillary bone

Occipital bone

Temporal bone

Sphenoid

Mandible

PLATE 6 A COMPUTER RECONSTRUCTION OF A DISARTICULATED SKULL

Optic canal

Anterior clinoid process

Superior orbital fissure

Foramen rotundum

Sella turcica

Posterior clinoid process

Foramen ovale

Foramen spinosum

Foramen lacerum

Petrous part of temporal bone

Internal acoustic canal

Jugular foramen

Crista galli of ethmoid

Anterior cranial fossa

Middle cranial fossa

Hypoglossal canal

Foramen magnum

Posterior cranial fossa

PLATE 7a THE CRANIAL FLOOR, DIAGRAMMATIC SUPERIOR VIEW

Anterior cranial fossa

Middle cranial fossa

Aqueduct of midbrain

Inferior colliculus

Posterior cranial fossa

Crista galli

Olfactory tract

Optic chiasm

Cerebral arterial circle

Cerebral peduncle

Superior colliculus

PLATE 7b THE CRANIAL FLOOR, SUPERIOR VIEW

PLATE **7c** THE CRANIAL
MENINGES, SUPERIOR VIEW

Loose connective
tissue and periosteum
of cranium

ANTERIOR

Cranium (skull)

Dura mater

Epicranial
aponeurosis

Subarachnoid
space

Scalp

Arachnoid
mater

Cerebral cortex
covered by
pia mater

POSTERIOR

PLATE **7d** DURAL FOLDS

Inferior
sagittal sinus

Falx cerebri

Superior
sagittal sinus

Optic nerve

Olfactory
tract

Frontal sinus

Crista galli

Olfactory
bulb

Third
ventricle

Tentorium
cerebelli

Cranium

Dura mater

Orbital process

Ethmoidal crest

Perpendicular plate

Conchal crest

Horizontal plate

Frontal process

Orbital rim

Maxillary sinus

Anterior nasal spine

Incisive canal

Palatal process

Alveolar process

PLATES **8a–b** PALATINE BONE, MEDIAL AND LATERAL VIEWS

PLATE **8c** RIGHT MAXILLARY BONE, MEDIAL VIEW

Maxillary bone eroded to show developing permanent teeth

Erupted primary teeth

First and second molars

Mandible eroded to show developing permanent teeth

PLATE **8d** MANDIBLE AND MAXILLARY BONES WITH UNERUPTED TEETH EXPOSED

Trochlear nerve (NIV)

Posterior cerebral artery

Cerebral peduncle

Inferior colliculus

Trigeminal nerve (V)

Superior

Middle

Cerebellar peduncles

Pons

Inferior

Facial (VII) and vestibulocochlear (VIII) nerves

Abducens nerve (VI)

Cerebellum

Roots of glossopharyngeal, vagus, and accessory nerves (IX, X, XI)

Root of hypoglossal nerve (XII)

Medulla oblongata

PLATE 9a BRAIN STEM, LATERAL VIEW

Superior colliculus

Inferior colliculus

Trochlear nerve (IV)

Cerebellar peduncles

Superior

Middle

Inferior

PLATE 9b BRAIN STEM, POSTERIOR VIEW

Corpora quadrigemina

Superior colliculi

Inferior colliculi

Trochlear nerve (IV)

Cerebral peduncle

Superior cerebellar peduncle

Reticular formation in floor of fourth ventricle

Fourth ventricle

PLATE 9c THE MESENCEPHALON, POSTERIOR VIEW

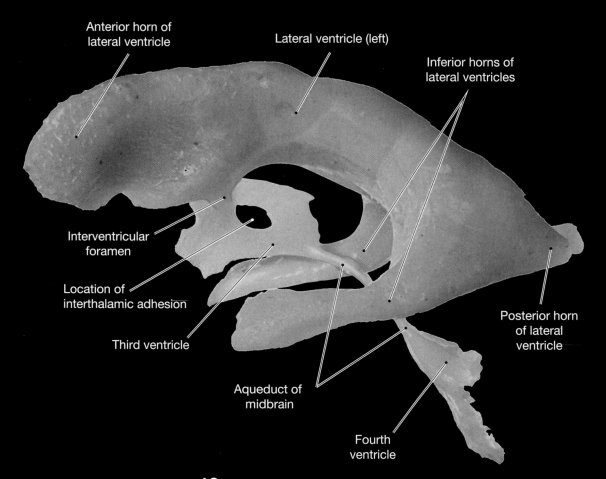

Anterior horn of
lateral ventricle

Lateral ventricle (left)

Inferior horns of
lateral ventricles

Interventricular
foramen

Location of
interthalamic adhesion

Third ventricle

Aqueduct of
midbrain

Fourth
ventricle

Posterior horn
of lateral
ventricle

PLATE **10** VENTRICLE CASTING, LATERAL VIEW

Cingulate gyrus

Lateral ventricle

Frontal lobe

Frontal sinus

Optic chiasm

Pituitary gland

Middle nasal concha

Sphenoidal sinus

Inferior nasal concha

Pons

Epiglottis

Trachea

Esophagus

Cranial meninges covering parietal lobe

Superior sagittal sinus

Corpus callosum

Fornix

Thalamus

Mamillary body

Corpora quadrigemina

Occipital lobe

Fourth ventricle

Cerebellum

Medulla oblongata

Margin of foramen magnum

Dura mater

Subarachnoid space

Spinal cord

PLATE **11a** MIDSAGITTAL SECTION THROUGH THE HEAD AND NECK

Cingulate gyrus

Frontal bone

Corpus callosum

Thalamus

Third ventricle

Mamillary body

Frontal sinus

Perpendicular plate of ethmoid

Optic nerve (II)

Cartilage of nasal septum

Vomer

Tongue

Genioglossus muscle

Mandible

Dens

Epiglottis

Mesencephalon

Pineal gland

Parietal bone

Colliculi

Superior

Inferior

Aqueduct of midbrain

Occipital bone

Cerebellum

Fourth ventricle

Transverse fibers of pons

Spinal cord

C₂

C₃

C₄

PLATE **11b** MRI SCAN OF THE BRAIN, MIDSAGITTAL SECTION

Longitudinal fissure

Corpus callosum

Caudate nucleus

Interventricular foramen

Putamen

Left thalamus

Globus pallidus

Third ventricle

Substantia nigra

Aqueduct of midbrain

Pons

Medulla oblongata

Lateral ventricles

Projection fibers of internal capsule

Insula

Septum pellucidum

Fornix

Temporal lobe

Cerebral peduncle

Cerebellum

Transverse fibers of pons

PLATE 11c **CORONAL SECTION THROUGH THE BRAIN AT THE LEVEL OF THE MESENCEPHALON AND PONS**

Cribriform plate of ethmoid

Medial rectus muscle

Optic nerve

Lateral rectus muscle

Ethmoidal labyrinth

Right internal carotid artery

Basilar artery

Mesencephalon

Cerebral peduncle

Cerebellum (anterior lobe)

Aqueduct of midbrain

Inferior sagittal sinus

Tentorium cerebelli

Tip of lateral ventricle

Occipital lobe of cerebrum

Superior sagittal sinus

Falx cerebri

PLATE 12a **HORIZONTAL SECTION THROUGH THE HEAD**

Septum pellucidum

Longitudinal fissure

Lateral ventricles

12b

Optic nerve (II)

Crista galli

Olfactory tracts

Inferior horn of lateral ventricle

Cerebral peduncles

Inferior colliculus

Cerebellum

Mesencephalon

Superior sagittal sinus

Aqueduct of midbrain

12c

Nasal septum

Maxillary sinus

Pyramids

External acoustic meatus

Olive

Medulla oblongata

Auricle

Cerebellar hemispheres

12d

PLATES **12b–d** MRI SCANS OF THE BRAIN, HORIZONTAL SECTIONS, SUPERIOR TO INFERIOR SEQUENCE

Lentiform
nucleus

Caudate
nucleus

Insula

Corpus
callosum

Lateral
ventricle

Septum
pellucidum

Fornix

Internal
capsule

Third
ventricle

Pineal
gland

Internal
capsule

Cerebellum

Lateral
ventricle

Thalamus

PLATE **13a** A HORIZONTAL SECTION THROUGH THE BRAIN

Longitudinal fissure
Lateral ventricle
Left frontal lobe
Sphenoidal sinus
Nasal septum
Temporal lobe
Inferior nasal concha
Masseter muscle

13b

Septum pellucidum
Corpus callosum
Superior sagittal sinus
Third ventricle
Interventricular foramen
Thalamus
Insula
Lateral sulcus
Temporal lobe

13c

Superior sagittal sinus
Septum pellucidum
Corpus callosum
Longitudinal fissure
Choroid plexus
Third ventricle
Lateral ventricle
Thalamus
Pons
Mesencephalon
Medulla oblongata
Spinal cord
Temporal lobe
Cerebellar peduncles

13d

Superior sagittal sinus
Cingulate gyrus
Corpus callosum
Longitudinal fissure
Lateral sulcus
Lateral ventricle
Choroid plexus
Fourth ventricle
Auricle
Cerebellum
Transverse sinus

13e

PLATES **13b–e** MRI SCANS OF THE BRAIN, FRONTAL (CORONAL) SECTIONS, ANTERIOR TO POSTERIOR SEQUENCE

Corpus
callosum

Longitudinal
fissure

Septum
pellucidum

Caudate
nucleus

Putamen

Clastrum

Insula

Left temporal
lobe

Lateral
ventricles

Internal
capsule

Right temporal
lobe

PLATE **13f** FRONTAL SECTION THROUGH THE BRAIN AT THE LEVEL OF THE BASAL NUCLEI

Maxillary
sinus

Cerebral
hemispheres

Crista
galli

Superior
nasal
concha

Middle
nasal
concha

Nasal
septum

Inferior
nasal
concha

PLATE **13g** MRI SCAN, CORONAL SECTION SHOWING PARANASAL SINUSES

Corpus callosum

Longitudinal fissure

Right cerebral hemisphere

A N T E R I O R

P O S T E R I O R

Cerebellum

Left cerebral hemisphere

Cerebral veins and arteries covered by arachnoid mater

PLATE **14a** SURFACE ANATOMY OF THE BRAIN, SUPERIOR VIEW

Longitudinal fissure

FRONTAL LOBE

Lateral fissure

TEMPORAL LOBE

Pons

Cerebellum

Medulla oblongata

PLATE **14b** SURFACE ANATOMY OF THE BRAIN, ANTERIOR VIEW

Longitudinal fssure

PARIETAL
LOBE

OCCIPITAL
LOBE

Left cerebral
hemisphere

Cerebellar
hemispheres

Medulla
oblongata

PLATE **14c** SURFACE ANATOMY OF THE BRAIN, POSTERIOR VIEW

Precentral gyrus

Central sulcus

FRONTAL
LOBE
(left cerebral hemisphere)

Postcentral
gyrus

PARIETAL LOBE

OCCIPITAL
LOBE

Lateral
sulcus

Branches of
middle cerebral
artery

Cerebellum

Pons

TEMPORAL
LOBE

Medulla
oblongata

PLATE **14d** SURFACE ANATOMY OF THE BRAIN, LATERAL VIEW

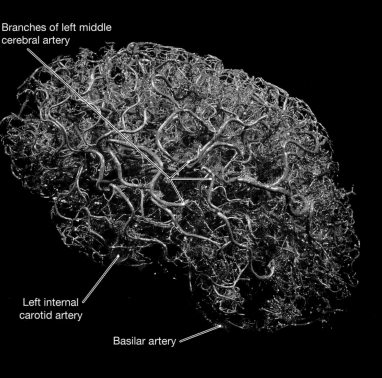

Branches of left middle
cerebral artery

Left internal
carotid artery

Basilar artery

PLATE 15a ARTERIAL CIRCULATION TO THE BRAIN, LATERAL VIEW OF CORROSION CAST

cerebral arteries

Anterior
communicating
artery

Posterior
communicating
artery

Posterior
cerebral artery

Left internal
carotid artery

Superior
cerebellar
artery

Pons

Basilar
artery

Anterior inferior
cerebellar artery

Vertebral
arteries

Medulla oblongata

PLATE 15c ARTERIES ON THE INFERIOR SURFACE OF THE BRAIN

Middle cerebral
artery

Anterior cerebral
artery

Internal carotid
artery

Levator palpebrae superioris muscle

Lacrimal gland

Eyeball

Superior oblique muscle

Superior rectus muscle

Trochlear nerve (IV)

Sensory branches of V

Abducens nerve (VI)

Optic nerve (II)

Lateral rectus muscle (reflected)

Internal carotid artery

Oculomotor nerve (III)

PLATES **16a–b** ACCESSORY STRUCTURES OF THE EYE, SUPERIOR VIEW

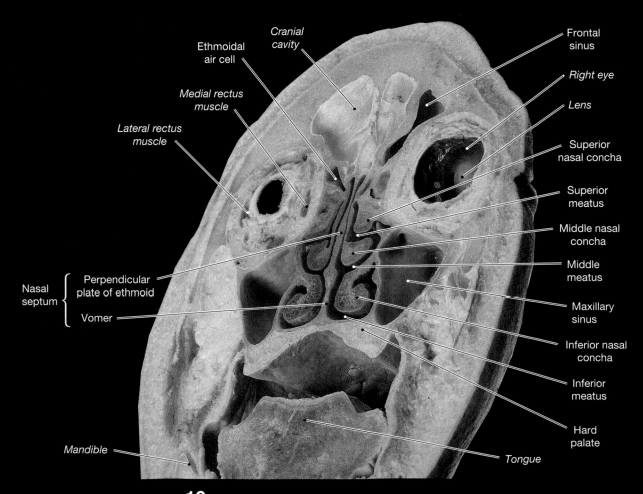

Cranial cavity

Ethmoidal air cell

Medial rectus muscle

Lateral rectus muscle

Nasal septum {
Perpendicular plate of ethmoid

Vomer
}

Mandible

Frontal sinus

Right eye

Lens

Superior nasal concha

Superior meatus

Middle nasal concha

Middle meatus

Maxillary sinus

Inferior nasal concha

Inferior meatus

Hard palate

Tongue

PLATE **16c** FRONTAL SECTION THROUGH THE FACE

Parietal region

Temporal region

Zygomatic arch

Angle of mandible

Anterior cervical triangle

External jugular vein

Clavicle

Occipital region

Mastoid process

Sternocleidomastoid muscle

Nuchal region

Trapezius muscle

Posterior cervical triangle

Acromion

Location of brachial plexus

PLATE 17 THE POSTERIOR CERVICAL TRIANGLE

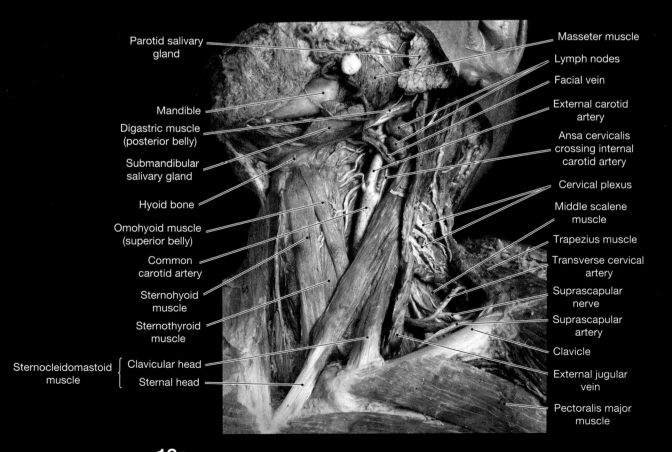

Parotid salivary gland

Mandible

Digastric muscle (posterior belly)

Submandibular salivary gland

Hyoid bone

Omohyoid muscle (superior belly)

Common carotid artery

Sternohyoid muscle

Sternothyroid muscle

Sternocleidomastoid muscle { Clavicular head / Sternal head

Masseter muscle

Lymph nodes

Facial vein

External carotid artery

Ansa cervicalis crossing internal carotid artery

Cervical plexus

Middle scalene muscle

Trapezius muscle

Transverse cervical artery

Suprascapular nerve

Suprascapular artery

Clavicle

External jugular vein

Pectoralis major muscle

PLATE 18a SUPERFICIAL STRUCTURES OF THE NECK, ANTEROLATERAL VIEW

Zygomatic arch

Temporalis muscle

Mandible (cut)

Styloglossus muscle

Lingual nerve

Sublingual salivary gland

Facial artery

Digastric muscle (anterior belly)

Hyoid bone

Superior thyroid artery

Common carotid artery

Sternohyoid muscle

Omohyoid muscle (superior belly)

Sternothyroid muscle

Thyroid gland

External carotid artery

Digastric muscle (posterior belly)

Great auricular nerve

Lesser occipital nerve

Splenius capitis muscle

Internal jugular vein

Cervical nerves

Trapezius muscle

Levator scapulae muscle

Ansa cervicalis

Middle scalene muscle

Clavicle

Omohyoid muscle (inferior belly)

PLATE **18b** DEEPER STRUCTURES OF THE NECK, LATERAL VIEW

Internal carotid artery

External carotid artery

Superior thyroid artery and vein

Common carotid artery

Inferior thyroid artery

Right clavicle (cut and removed)

Thyrocervical trunk

Subclavian artery

Subclavian vein

Brachiocephalic trunk

Right brachiocephalic vein

Thyroid cartilage

Cricoid cartilage

Internal jugular vein

Thyroid gland

Inferior thyroid veins

Manubrium of sternum (cut)

Left brachiocephalic vein

PLATE **18c** DEEPER STRUCTURES OF THE NECK, ANTERIOR VIEW

Arbor vitae of cerebellum

Foramen magnum

Inferior nasal concha

Choroid plexus

Hard palate

Soft palate

External occipital crest

Nasopharynx

Dens of axis

Tongue

Uvula

(C₂)

Atlas (C₁) (anterior arch)

Oropharynx

C₃

Mandible

Atlas (C₁) (posterior arch)

Epiglottis

C₄

Hyoid bone

Laryngopharynx

C₅

Ventricular fold

Vocal fold

Spinal cord

C₆

Thyroid cartilage

Spinous processes of vertebrae

C₇

Cricoid cartilage

T₁

Tracheal cartilages

Esophagus

T₂

External jugular vein

Trachea

Right common carotid artery

T₃

Aortic arch

Manubrium of sternum

Left brachiocephalic vein

Pleural cavity

Body of sternum

PLATE **19** MIDSAGITTAL SECTION THROUGH THE HEAD AND NECK

Cervical
spinal cord

Rootlets
of C_8

Dorsal root
ganglion of C_8

Dura mater

Dorsal root
ganglia of T_4
and T_5

PLATE 20a THE CERVICAL AND
THORACIC REGIONS OF THE SPINAL
CORD, POSTERIOR VIEW

Pons

Fourth
ventricle

Medulla
oblongata

Dens
of axis

Longus
capitis muscle

C_2 (axis)

Intervertebral
disc

C_3

T_1

Arbor
vitae of
cerebellum

Posterior
arch of
C_1 (atlas)

Trapezius
muscle

Semispinalis
capitis muscle

Semispinalis
cervicis muscle

Spinous
process
of C_7
(vertebra
prominens)

Dura
mater

Spinal
cord

PLATE 20b MRI SCAN OF CERVICAL REGION, SAGITTAL SECTION

Facet for dens
Posterior tubercle
Posterior arch
Transverse foramen

Verbebral foramen

Superior articular process
Superior articular facet
Anterior tubercle
Anterior arch
Costal process
Transverse process

PLATE 21a ATLAS, SUPERIOR VIEW

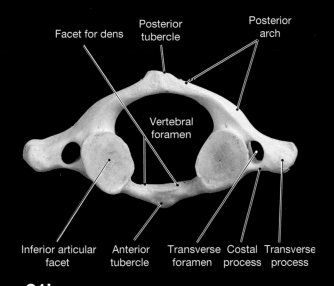

Facet for dens
Posterior tubercle
Posterior arch

Vertebral foramen

Inferior articular facet
Anterior tubercle
Transverse foramen
Costal process
Transverse process

PLATE 21b ATLAS, INFERIOR VIEW

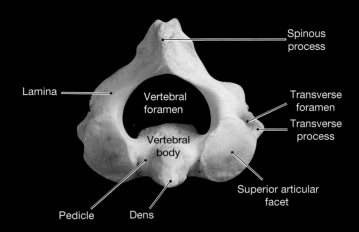

Spinous process

Lamina
Vertebral foramen
Transverse foramen
Transverse process

Vertebral body

Pedicle
Dens
Superior articular facet

PLATE 21c AXIS, SUPERIOR VIEW

Spinous process

Lamina

Inferior articular process

Inferior articular facet

Transverse process

Vertebral foramen

Vertebral body

Transverse foramen
Superior articular process
Pedicle

PLATE 21d AXIS, INFERIOR VIEW

Articular facet for dens of axis

Dens

Atlas (C1)

Axis (C2)

PLATE 21e ARTICULATED ATLAS AND AXIS, SUPERIOR AND POSTERIOR VIEW

Superior articular facet

Transverse process

Lamina

Spinous process

PLATE **22a** THORACIC VERTEBRA, POSTERIOR VIEW

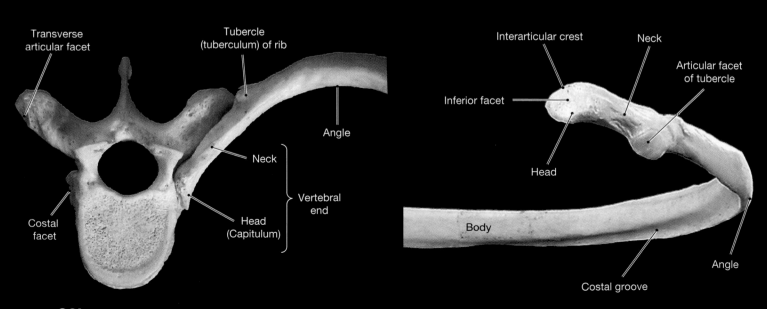

Transverse articular facet

Tubercle (tuberculum) of rib

Angle

Neck

Vertebral end

Costal facet

Head (Capitulum)

Interarticular crest

Neck

Articular facet of tubercle

Inferior facet

Head

Body

Angle

Costal groove

PLATE **22b** THORACIC VERTEBRA AND RIB, SUPERIOR VIEW

PLATE **22c** REPRESENTATIVE RIB, POSTERIOR VIEW

Spinous process

Superior
articular
process

Transverse
process

Vertebral
body

Inferior articular
facet

Pedicle

PLATE 23a THE LUMBAR VERTEBRAE, LATERAL VIEW

Lamina

Spinous
process

Superior
articular
facet

Transverse
process

Superior
articular process

Pedicle

Vertebral
foramen

Vertebral
body

PLATE 23b THE LUMBAR VERTEBRAE, SUPERIOR VIEW

Vertebral body

Intervertebral
disc

Compression
fracture

Spinous
process

Transverse
process

PLATE 23c 3-DIMENSIONAL CT SCAN SHOWING A FRACTURE
OF THE BODY OF A LUMBAR VERTEBRA

Conus medullaris
of spinal cord

Cauda equina

Dura mater

Dorsal root
ganglia of L_2
and L_3

1st sacral
nerve root

Sacrum (cut)

Filum terminale

PLATE 24a THE INFERIOR PORTION OF THE
VERTEBRAL COLUMN, POSTERIOR VIEW

Spinal cord

L_5 vertebra

Filum terminale

Subarachnoid space
containing cerebrospinal
fluid and spinal nerve roots

Terminal portion
of filum terminale

S_2 vertebra

PLATE 24b MRI SCAN OF INFERIOR PORTION OF THE
VERTEBRAL CANAL, LATERAL VIEW

L_4 Vertebra

L_5 Vertebra

Cauda
equina

PLATE 24c X-RAY OF THE CAUDA EQUINA WITH A
CONTRAST MEDIUM IN THE SUBARACHNOID SPACE

Dura mater

Epidural space

Body of 3rd
lumbar vertebra

Interspinous
ligament

Lumbar puncture
needle

Cauda equina in
subarachnoid space

Filum terminale

PLATE 24d LUMBAR PUNCTURE POSITIONING, SEEN IN A
SAGITTAL SECTION

Zygomaticus minor muscle

Zygomaticus major muscle

Oribicularis oris muscle

Omohyoid muscle

Sternohyoid muscle

Sternocleidomastoid muscle

Cephalic
vein

Superclavicular
nerves

Pectoralis
major muscle
(clavicular head)

Pectoralis
major muscle
(sternocostal head)

PLATE 25 SHOULDER AND NECK, ANTERIOR VIEW

Acromioclavicular
joint

Scapula

Sternoclavicular
joint

Manubrium
of sternum

Clavicle

PLATE **26a** BONES OF THE RIGHT PECTORAL GIRDLE, SUPERIOR VIEW

Anterior sternoclavicular
ligament

Interclavicular
ligament

Sternal end
of clavicle

Manubrium
of sternum

1st rib

Clavicle

Subclavius
muscle

Costoclavicular
ligament

Costal
cartilages

2nd rib

PLATE **26b** STERNOCLAVICULAR JOINT

Acromial end of clavicle

Deltoid muscle

Teres major muscle

Triceps brachii muscle, long head

Triceps brachii muscle, lateral head

Lateral epicondyle of humerus

Olecranon

Anconeus muscle

Extensor digitorum muscle

Head of ulna

Biceps brachii muscle

Brachialis muscle

Tendon of biceps brachii

Brachioradialis muscle

Extensor carpi radialis longus muscle

Extensor carpi radialis brevis muscle

Styloid process of radius

PLATE **27a** RIGHT UPPER LIMB AND TRUNK, LATERAL VIEW

Vertebral border of scapula

Teres major muscle

Inferior angle of scapula

Triceps brachii muscle, long head

Triceps brachii muscle, medial head

Tendon of insertion of triceps brachii

Medial epicondyle of humerus

Site of palpation for ulnar nerve

Olecranon

Anconeus muscle

Extensor carpi ulnaris muscle

Flexor carpi ulnaris muscle

Spine of scapula

Infraspinatus muscle

Site of axillary nerve

Triceps brachii muscle, lateral head

Brachioradialis muscle

Extensor carpi radialis longus muscle

Extensor carpi radialis brevis muscle

Extensor digitorum muscle

PLATE **27b** RIGHT UPPER LIMB AND TRUNK, POSTERIOR VIEW

Deltoid muscle

Cephalic vein

Biceps brachii
muscle

Cephalic vein

Brachioradialis
muscle

Median antebrachial
vein

Pectoralis major
muscle

Coracobrachialis
muscle

Triceps brachii
muscle, long head

Basilic vein

Median cubital vein

PLATE 27c RIGHT ARM AND TRUNK, ANTERIOR VIEW

Head of
humerus

Deltoid
muscle

Infraspinatus
muscle

Subscapularis
muscle

Glenoid
cavity

Glenoid
labrum

Articular
capsule

Axillary
vein

Pectoralis
major
muscle

Cephalic
vein

Greater
tubercle

Intertubercular
groove

Lesser
tubercle

**PLATE 27d HORIZONTAL SECTION THROUGH THE RIGHT
SHOULDER**

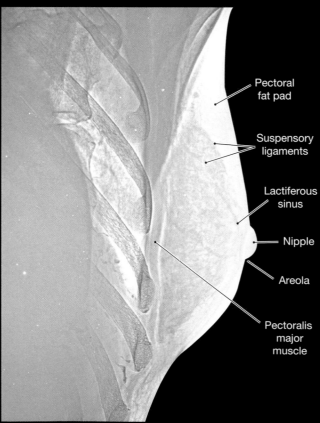

Pectoral
fat pad

Suspensory
ligaments

Lactiferous
sinus

Nipple

Areola

Pectoralis
major
muscle

PLATE 28 XEROMAMMOGRAM

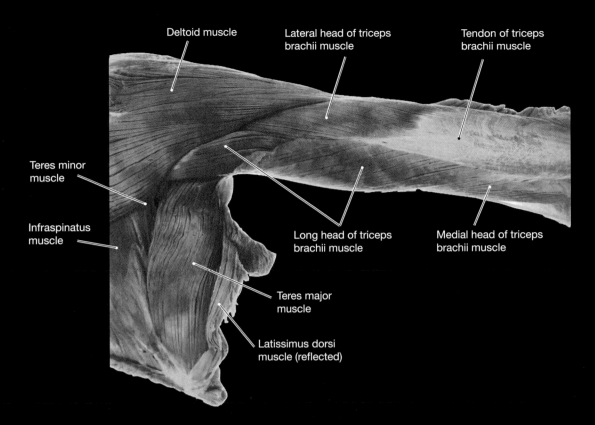

Deltoid muscle

Lateral head of triceps brachii muscle

Tendon of triceps brachii muscle

Teres minor muscle

Infraspinatus muscle

Long head of triceps brachii muscle

Medial head of triceps brachii muscle

Teres major muscle

Latissimus dorsi muscle (reflected)

PLATE **29a** SUPERFICIAL DISSECTION OF RIGHT SHOULDER, POSTERIOR VIEW

Deltoid muscle

Median nerve

Axillary nerve

Musculocutaneous nerve

Coracobrachialis muscle

Biceps brachii muscle

Pectoralis minor muscle

Long head of triceps brachii muscle

Lateral cord

Posterior cord

Lateral head of triceps brachii muscle

Medial cord

Medial head of triceps brachii muscle

Medial brachial cutaneous nerve

Thoracodorsal nerve

Subscapularis muscle

Medial antebrachial cutaneous nerve

Ulnar nerve

Teres major muscle

Latissimus dorsi muscle

PLATE **29b** DEEP DISSECTION OF THE RIGHT BRACHIAL PLEXUS

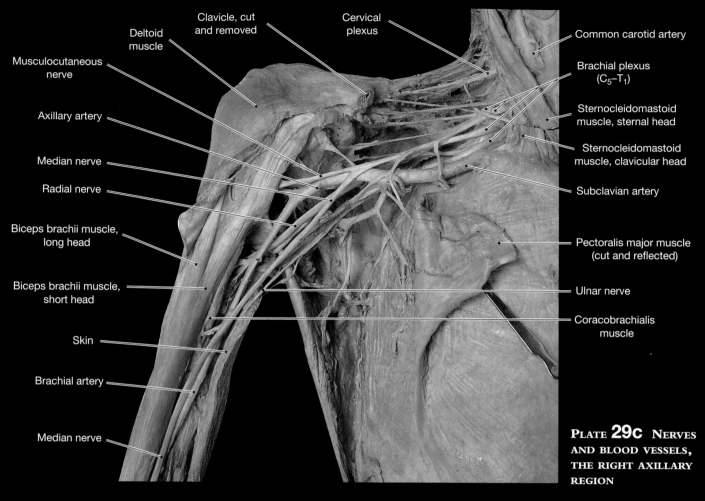

Clavicle, cut and removed

Cervical plexus

Common carotid artery

Deltoid muscle

Brachial plexus (C₅–T₁)

Musculocutaneous nerve

Sternocleidomastoid muscle, sternal head

Axillary artery

Sternocleidomastoid muscle, clavicular head

Median nerve

Subclavian artery

Radial nerve

Biceps brachii muscle, long head

Pectoralis major muscle (cut and reflected)

Biceps brachii muscle, short head

Ulnar nerve

Skin

Coracobrachialis muscle

Brachial artery

Median nerve

PLATE 29C NERVES AND BLOOD VESSELS, THE RIGHT AXILLARY REGION

Biceps brachii muscle

Brachioradialis muscle

Brachial artery

Inferior ulnar collateral artery

Ulnar artery

Radial artery

Radial artery

Pronator teres muscle

Palmaris longus muscle

Flexor carpi ulnaris muscle

Flexor carpi radialis muscle

Ulnar artery

Superficial palmar arch

PLATE 30 NERVES AND BLOOD VESSELS, THE RIGHT ARM AND FOREARM

Scapula

Humerus

Radius

Ulna

Carpal bones

Metacarpal
bones (I to V)

Phalanges

Os coxae (hip bone)

Femur

Patella

Tibia

Fibula

Tarsal bones

Metatarsal bones

Phalanges

PLATE **31** BONES OF THE RIGHT UPPER LIMB, ANTERIOR
VIEW

PLATE **32** BONES OF THE RIGHT LOWER LIMB, LATERAL
VIEW

Triceps brachii muscle, long head

Biceps brachii muscle

Triceps brachii muscle, medial head

Triceps brachii muscle, lateral head

Brachialis muscle

Brachioradialis muscle

Medial epicondyle of humerus

Biceps brachii muscle

Brachialis muscle

Median nerve

Brachioradialis muscle

Pronator teres muscle

Flexor carpi radialis muscle

Palmaris longus muscle

Tendon of palmaris longus

PLATE **33a** THE RIGHT UPPER LIMB, ANTERIOR SURFACE, MUSCLES

PLATE **33b** THE RIGHT UPPER LIMB, ANTERIOR VIEW, SUPERFICIAL DISSECTION

Acromion

Deltoid muscle

Triceps brachii muscle, long head

Triceps brachii muscle, lateral head

Olecranon of ulna

Flexor carpi ulnaris muscle

Extensor carpi radialis longus muscle

Extensor carpi radialis brevis muscle

Extensor carpi ulnaris muscle

Extensor digitorum muscle

Deltoid muscle

Teres major muscle

Triceps brachii muscle, long head

Latissimus dorsi muscle

Triceps brachii muscle, lateral head

Flexor carpi ulnaris muscle

Palmaris longus muscle

Flexor digitorum superficialis muscle

Flexor digitorum profundus muscle

Flexor carpi ulnaris muscle

Ulna

Tendon of extensor carpi ulnaris

Tendon of flexor carpi radialis

Flexor retinaculum

Tendon of palmaris longus

Extensor retinaculum

PLATE **33c** THE RIGHT UPPER LIMB, POSTERIOR SURFACE, LANDMARKS

PLATE **33d** THE RIGHT UPPER LIMB, POSTERIOR VIEW, SUPERFICIAL DISSECTION

Intertubercular groove

Lesser tubercle

Head

Greater tubercle

Anatomical neck

Surgical neck

Intertubercular groove

Shaft (body)

Deltoid tuberosity

Coronoid fossa

Radial fossa

Lateral epicondyle

Medial epicondyle

Capitulum

Trochlea

Condyle

Head

Greater tubercle

Anatomical neck

Surgical neck

Deltoid tuberosity

Radial groove for radial nerve

Olecranon fossa

Lateral epicondyle

Medial epicondyle

Trochlea

PLATE 34a RIGHT HUMERUS, ANTERIOR VIEW

PLATE 34b RIGHT HUMERUS, POSTERIOR VIEW

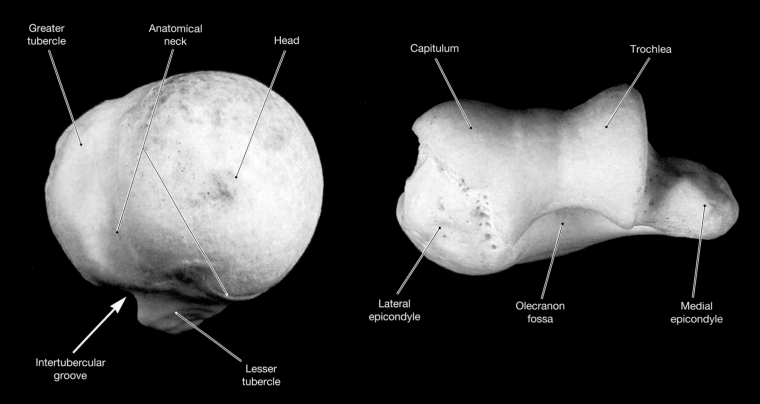

Greater tubercle

Anatomical neck

Head

Intertubercular groove

Lesser tubercle

Capitulum

Trochlea

Lateral epicondyle

Olecranon fossa

Medial epicondyle

PLATE 34c PROXIMAL END OF RIGHT HUMERUS, SUPERIOR VIEW

PLATE 34d DISTAL END OF RIGHT HUMERUS, INFERIOR VIEW

Humerus

Olecranon fossa

Medial epicondyle of humerus

Olecranon

Capitulum of humerus

Head of radius

Ulna

PLATE 35a RIGHT ELBOW JOINT, POSTERIOR VIEW

Humerus

Medial epicondyle

Trochlea

Capitulum

Head of radius

Radial notch of ulna

Coronoid process of ulna

PLATE 35b RIGHT ELBOW JOINT, ANTERIOR VIEW

Radius

Ulna

Head of
radius

Capitulum

Trochlea

Humerus
(cut edge
of shaft)

Medial
epicondyle

PLATE 35c 3-DIMENSIONAL CT SCAN OF THE RIGHT
ELBOW JOINT, SUPERIOR VIEW

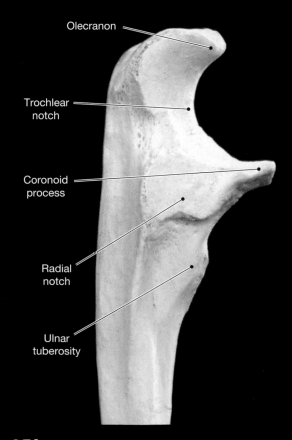

Medial
epicondyle
of humerus

Capitulum of
humerus

Trochlea of
humerus

Annular
ligament

Articular
capsule

Head of
radius

Coronoid
process
of ulna

Radial notch
of ulna

Trochlear notch
of ulna

Olecranon

PLATE 35e ARTICULAR SURFACES WITHIN THE RIGHT
ELBOW JOINT

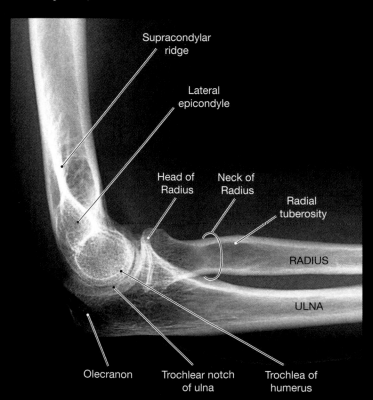

Supracondylar
ridge

Lateral
epicondyle

Head of
Radius

Neck of
Radius

Radial
tuberosity

RADIUS

ULNA

Olecranon

Trochlear notch
of ulna

Trochlea of
humerus

PLATE 35d X-RAY OF THE ELBOW JOINT, MEDIAL-LATERAL
PROJECTION

Olecranon

Trochlear
notch

Coronoid
process

Radial
notch

Ulnar
tuberosity

PLATE 35f RIGHT ULNA, LATERAL VIEW

Humerus

Triceps
brachii
muscle

Tendon
of triceps
brachii

Articular
cartilage of
olecranon

Bursa

Articular
cartilage
of radius

Ulnar
artery

Flexor
digitorum
profundus
muscle

Biceps
brachii
muscle

Brachialis
muscle

Radial
artery

Articular
capsule

Joint
cavity

Articular
cartilage of
capitulum

Pronator
teres
muscle

Flexor
digitorum
superficialis
muscle

PLATE 35g THE ELBOW, OBLIQUE SECTION—MODEL

Olecranon

Coronoid
process

Trochlear
notch

Radial notch
of ulna

Head of radius

Neck of radius

Ulnar
tuberosity

Radial
tuberosity

ULNA

RADIUS

Attachment
surfaces for
interosseous
membrane

Ulnar notch
of radius

Head of ulna

Distal radioulnar
joint

Ulnar styloid
process

Radial
styloid process

Carpal
articular surface

Olecranon

Proximal radioulnar
joint

Head of
radius

Neck of
radius

RADIUS

ULNA

Ulnar notch
of radius

Ulnar
head

Ulnar
styloid
process

Radial
styloid
process

Distal extremity
of radius

PLATE **36a** RIGHT RADIUS AND ULNA, ANTERIOR VIEW   PLATE **36b** RIGHT RADIUS AND ULNA, POSTERIOR VIEW

Cephalic vein over biceps brachii muscle

Cephalic vein

Tendon of palmaris longus

Tendon of flexor carpi radialis

Site for palpation of radial pulse

Median cubital vein

Cubital fossa

Median antebrachial vein

Flexor digitorum superficialis muscle

Flexor carpi ulnaris muscle

Head of ulna

Pisiform bone

PLATE 37a THE RIGHT UPPER LIMB, ANTERIOR SURFACE, LANDMARKS

Tendon of extensor carpi radialis longus

Tendon of extensor pollicis brevis

Extensor pollicis longus muscle

Tendon of extensor carpi radialis longus

Tendon of extensor carpi radialis brevis

Extensor pollicis brevis muscle

Abductor pollicis longus muscle

Extensor carpi radialis brevis muscle

Extensor carpi radialis longus muscle

First dorsal interosseus muscle

Tendons of extensor indicis

Abductor digiti minimi muscle

Brachioradialis muscle

Tendons of extensor digitorum

Tendons of extensor digiti minimi

Tendons of extensor carpi radialis brevis

Extensor retinaculum

Extensor muscle

Extensor digitorum muscle

Extensor digiti minimi muscle

Extensor carpi ulnaris muscle

PLATE 37b SUPERFICIAL DISSECTION OF LEFT FOREARM AND HAND, POSTERIOR VIEW

Radius

Ulna

Scaphoid

Lunate

Capitate

Pisiform

Triquetrum

Trapezium

Hamate

Trapezoid

I   II   III   IV   V

PLATE **38a** BONES OF THE RIGHT WRIST, ANTERIOR VIEW

Ulnar
collateral
ligament

Radiocarpal
articulation

Carpometacarpal
articulations

Radial collateral
ligament

Intercarpal
articulations

Collateral
ligaments

I

V   IV   III   II

Interphalangeal
articulations

Metacarpophalangeal
articulations

PLATE **38b** JOINTS OF THE RIGHT WRIST, CORONAL
SECTION

PLATE **38c** THE RIGHT HAND, POSTERIOR VIEW—MODEL

Tendon of extensor indicis

Tendon of extensor pollicis longus

Digital nerve

Dorsal digital arteries

Collateral ligament

Interphalangeal joint

Tendon of extensor digiti minimi

Radial artery

Tendons of extensor digitorum

Tendon of extensor carpi radialis longus

Abductor digiti minimi muscle

Dorsal interosseus muscles

Tendon of extensor carpi radialis brevis

Extensor retinaculum

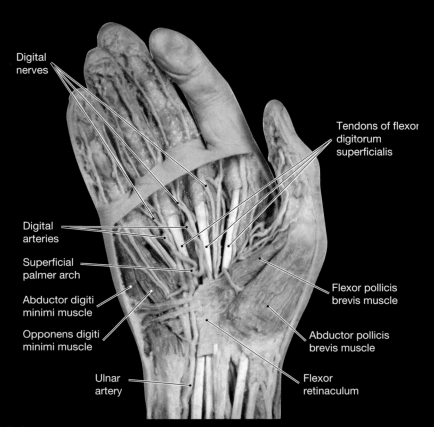

Digital nerves

Tendons of flexor digitorum superficialis

Digital arteries

Superficial palmer arch

Abductor digiti minimi muscle

Opponens digiti minimi muscle

Flexor pollicis brevis muscle

Abductor pollicis brevis muscle

Ulnar artery

Flexor retinaculum

PLATE **38d** SUPERFICIAL DISSECTION OF THE RIGHT WRIST AND HAND, ANTERIOR VIEW

Tendon of flexor digitorum profundus

Tendon of flexor digitorum superficialis

Synovial sheaths

Lumbrical muscle

Tendon of flexor pollicis longus

Tendons of flexor digitorum

Superficial palmar arch

Abductor digiti minimi muscle

Flexor pollicis brevis muscle

Flexor digiti minimi muscle

Abductor pollicis brevis muscle

Palmaris brevis muscle

Flexor retinaculum

Ulnar nerve

Tendon of palmaris longus

Tendon of flexor carpi radialis

Flexor digitorum superficialis muscle

Radial artery

Flexor carpi ulnaris muscle

Ulnar artery

Median nerve

PLATE 38e   THE RIGHT HAND, ANTERIOR VIEW, SUPERFICIAL DISSECTION

Lumbrical muscles

Abductor pollicis muscle

Tendon of flexor pollicis longus

Abductor digiti minimi muscle

Flexor pollicis brevis muscle

Flexor digiti minimi muscle

Abductor pollicis brevis muscle

Ulnar artery

Tendon of abductor pollicis longus

Tendons of flexor digitorum superficialis

Tendon of flexor carpi radialis

PLATE 38f   FLEXOR TENDONS OF RIGHT WRIST AND HAND

Jugular notch

Clavicle

Acromion

Manubrium of sternum

Body of sternum

Axilla

Xiphoid process

Costal margin of ribs

Median cubital vein

Medial epicondyle

Sternocleidomastoid muscle

Anterior edge of trapezius muscle

Posterior cervical triangle

Deltoid muscle

Pectoralis major muscle

Areola and nipple

Biceps brachii muscle

Linea alba

Umbilicus

PLATE **39a** SURFACE ANATOMY OF THE TRUNK, ANTERIOR VIEW

Xiphoid process

Rectus abdominis muscle

Umbilicus

Anterior superior iliac spine

Inguinal ligament

Inguinal canal

Tendinous inscriptions of rectus abdominis

Serratus anterior muscle

Latissimus dorsi muscle

External oblique muscle

Pubic symphysis

PLATE **39b** SURFACE ANATOMY OF THE ABDOMEN, ANTERIOR VIEW

Sternocleidomastoid
muscle

Sternohyoid muscle

Sternothyroid muscle

Deltoid muscle
(anterior fibers)

External
intercostal
muscles

Pectoralis
minor muscle

Pectoralis
major muscle

Serratus anterior
muscle

Rectus abdominis
muscle

External oblique
muscle

Latissimus dorsi
muscle

Tendinous inscriptions

Linea alba

External
oblique
aponeurosis

PLATE **39c** TRUNK, ANTERIOR VIEW

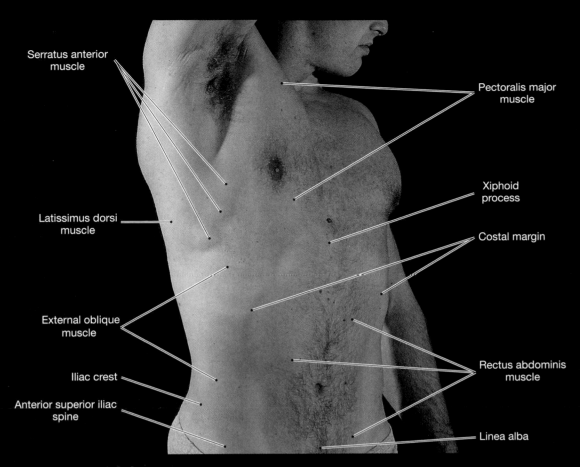

Serratus anterior muscle

Pectoralis major muscle

Latissimus dorsi muscle

Xiphoid process

Costal margin

External oblique muscle

Iliac crest

Rectus abdominis muscle

Anterior superior iliac spine

Linea alba

PLATE **39d** SURFACE ANATOMY OF THE ABDOMEN, ANTEROLATERAL VIEW

Acromion

Triceps brachii muscle, lateral head

Biceps brachii muscle

Triceps brachii muscle, long head

Deltoid muscle

Vertebra prominens (C$_7$)

Spine of scapula

Infraspinatus muscle

Vertebral border of scapula

Trapezius muscle

Teres major muscle

Inferior angle of scapula

Latissimus dorsi muscle

Erector spinae muscles

PLATE **40a** SURFACE ANATOMY OF THE TRUNK, POSTERIOR VIEW

Deltoid muscle
(posterior fibers)

Rhomboid minor muscle

Rhomboid major muscle

Triceps brachii muscle

Infraspinatus
muscle

Latissimus dorsi muscle

Lumbodorsal (thoracolumbar)
fascia

Gluteus medius muscle

Gluteus maximus muscle

PLATE **40b** TRUNK, POSTERIOR VIEW

Serratus anterior muscle

Tendinous inscription

Rectus abdominis muscle

External oblique muscle

Umbilicus

PLATE **41a** ABDOMINAL WALL, ANTERIOR VIEW

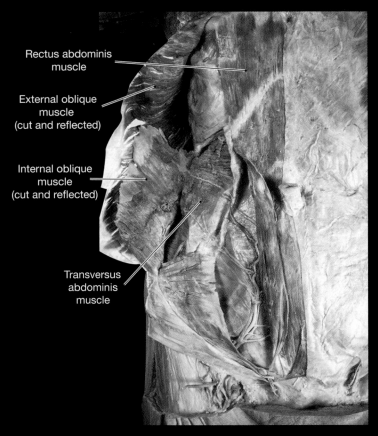

Rectus abdominis muscle

External oblique muscle (cut and reflected)

Internal oblique muscle (cut and reflected)

Transversus abdominis muscle

PLATE **41b** ABDOMINAL MUSCLES

Right subclavian artery

Right common carotid artery

Brachiocephalic trunk

Left brachiocephalic vein

Trachea

Superior lobe, right lung

Left primary bronchus

Superior vena cava

Superior lobe, left lung

Pulmonary trunk

Right primary bronchus

Pulmonary arteries

Left ventricle

Pulmonary veins

Anterior interventricular artery

Middle lobe, right lung

Inferior lobe, left lung

Right atrium

Marginal branch of right coronary artery

Apex of heart

Inferior lobe, right lung

Right ventricle

PLATE 42a   THE HEART AND LUNGS, ANTERIOR VIEW

Apical

Apical and posterior (fused)

Superior lobe

Posterior

Superior lobe

Anterior

Anterior

Superior lingular

Inferior lingular

Middle lobe

Lateral

Medial

Superior

Inferior lobe

Superior

Anterior basal

Anterior basal

Medial basal

Lateral basal

Inferior lobe

Lateral basal

Posterior basal

Posterior basal

Medial basal

PLATE 42b   COLOR-CODED CORROSION CAST OF THE BRONCHIAL TREE, ANTERIOR VIEW

Apex of
right lung

Apex of
left lung

Right primary
bronchus

Trachea

Aortic arch

Right superior
lobar bronchus

Left primary
bronchus

Right middle
lobar bronchus

Left superior
lobar bronchus

Right inferior
lobar bronchus

Left inferior
lobar bronchus

Diaphragm

PLATE 42c COLORIZED BRONCHOGRAM 1

Catheter
within
trachea

Ribs

Right
primary
bronchus

*Left
primary
bronchus*

Secondary
bronchi

PLATE 42d COLORIZED BRONCHOGRAM 2

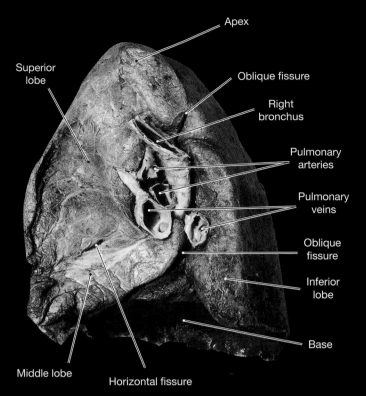

Apex

Superior lobe

Oblique fissure

Right bronchus

Pulmonary arteries

Pulmonary veins

Oblique fissure

Inferior lobe

Base

Middle lobe

Horizontal fissure

PLATE **43a** MEDIAL SURFACE OF RIGHT LUNG

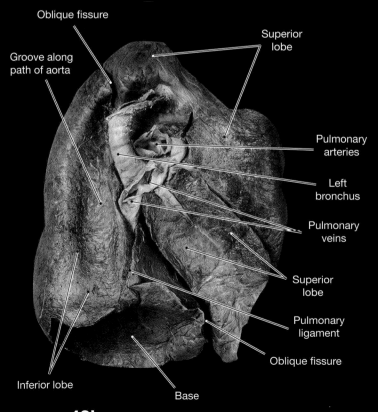

Oblique fissure

Superior lobe

Groove along path of aorta

Pulmonary arteries

Left bronchus

Pulmonary veins

Superior lobe

Pulmonary ligament

Oblique fissure

Inferior lobe

Base

PLATE **43b** MEDIAL SURFACE OF LEFT LUNG

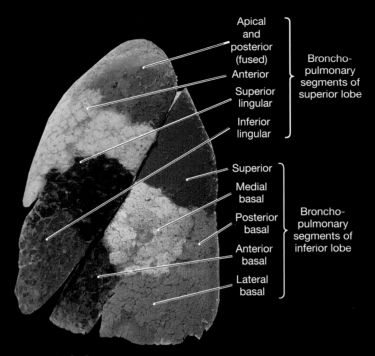

Bronchopulmonary segments of superior lobe { Apical / Posterior / Anterior

Bronchopulmonary segments of middle lobe { Medial / Lateral

Bronchopulmonary segments of inferior lobe { Superior / Lateral basal / Posterior basal / Anterior basal

Apical and posterior (fused) / Anterior / Superior lingular / Inferior lingular } Bronchopulmonary segments of superior lobe

Superior / Medial basal / Posterior basal / Anterior basal / Lateral basal } Bronchopulmonary segments of inferior lobe

PLATE **43c** BRONCHOPULMONARY SEGMENTS IN THE RIGHT LUNG, LATERAL VIEW

PLATE **43d** BRONCHOPULMONARY SEGMENTS IN THE LEFT LUNG, LATERAL VIEW

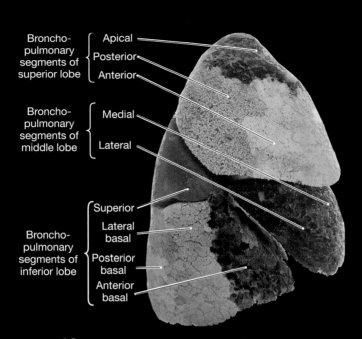

Apical

Anterior

Lateral

Medial

Lateral

Medial

Lateral

Anterior basal

Medial basal

Posterior basal

Lateral basal

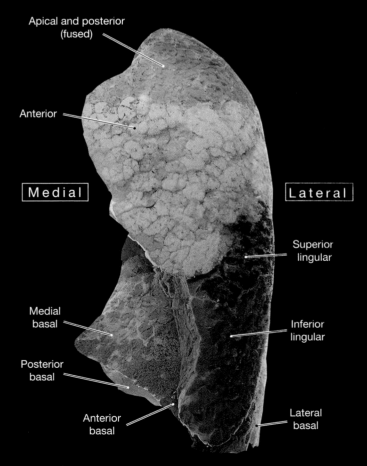

Apical and posterior (fused)

Anterior

Medial

Lateral

Superior lingular

Medial basal

Posterior basal

Inferior lingular

Anterior basal

Lateral basal

PLATE **44a** BRONCHOPULMONARY SEGMENTS IN THE RIGHT LUNG, ANTERIOR VIEW

PLATE **44b** BRONCHOPULMONARY SEGMENTS IN THE LEFT LUNG, ANTERIOR VIEW

Catheter for dye injection, passing through the right atrium and right ventricle to the pulmonary trunk

Right pulmonary artery

Right atrium

Right ventricle

Left pulmonary artery

Pulmonary trunk

Left ventricle

PLATE **44c** PULMONARY ANGIOGRAM

Right common carotid artery

Right vertebral artery

Right subclavian artery

Right internal thoracic artery

Brachiocephalic trunk

Left common carotid artery

Left vertebral artery

Left axillary artery

Left subclavian artery

Aortic arch

Descending thoracic aorta

PLATE **45a** AORTIC ANGIOGRAM

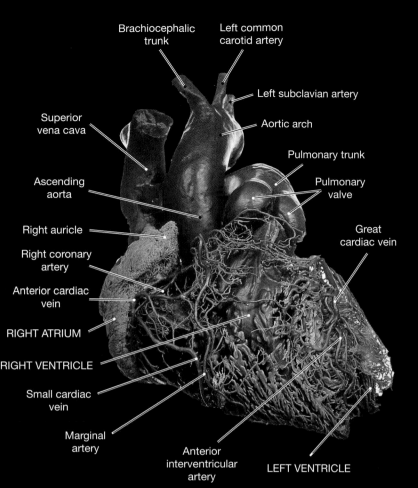

Brachiocephalic trunk

Left common carotid artery

Left subclavian artery

Aortic arch

Superior vena cava

Pulmonary trunk

Pulmonary valve

Ascending aorta

Great cardiac vein

Right auricle

Right coronary artery

Anterior cardiac vein

RIGHT ATRIUM

RIGHT VENTRICLE

Small cardiac vein

Marginal artery

Anterior interventricular artery

LEFT VENTRICLE

Right coronary artery

Right marginal artery

Left coronary artery

Circumflex artery

Left marginal artery

Anterior interventricular artery

Apex of heart

PLATE **45c** CORONARY ANGIOGRAM, LATERAL VIEW

Left atrium

Left AV
(bicuspid) valve

*Inferior
vena cava*

Chordae
tendineae

Papillary
muscle of left
ventricle

Pectinate
muscles

Interventricular
septum

Trabeculae carneae
of right ventricle

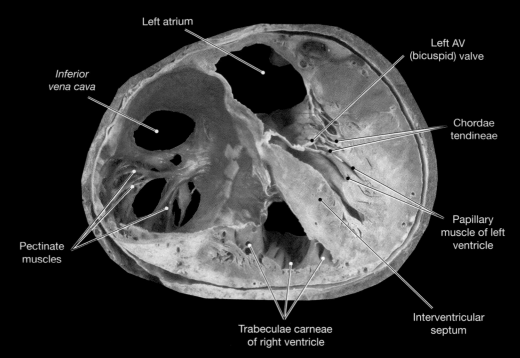

PLATE 45d HORIZONTAL SECTION THROUGH THE HEART, SUPERIOR VIEW

Pericardium (cut)

Costal cartilage

Esophagus

Diaphragm

Left phrenic nerve

Pleural space

Central tendon of
diaphragm

Thoracic aorta

Spinal cord

Intervertebral disc
of thoracic vertebra

Inferior vena cava

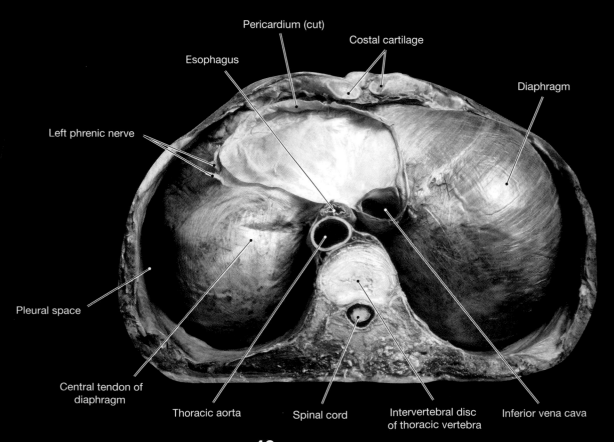

PLATE 46 DIAPHRAGM, SUPERIOR VIEW

Sternocleidomastoid muscle

Omohyoid, sternothyroid and sternohyoid muscles

Right common carotid artery

Subclavian vein

Right axillary artery

Right axillary vein

Superior vena cava

Right lung, superior lobe

Horizontal fissure

Right lung, middle lobe

Oblique fissure

Right lung, inferior lobe

Diaphragm

Right lobe of liver

Left common carotid artery

Anterior scalene muscle

Thyroid gland

Thyrocervical trunk

Clavicle, cut

Trachea

Thymus

Left lung, superior lobe

Left lung, inferior lobe

Left lobe of liver

PLATE **47a** THORACIC ORGANS, SUPERFICIAL VIEW—MODEL

Trachea

Right lung, superior lobe

Superior vena cava

Right superior lobar bronchus

Right pulmonary arteries and veins

Right middle lobar bronchus

Right lung, middle lobe

Right inferior lobar bronchus

Right lung, inferior lobe

Right and left ventricles

Left external carotid artery

Left internal carotid artery

Carotid sinus

Left internal jugular vein

Left subclavian vein

Left brachiocephalic vein

Left lung, superior lobe

Aortic arch

Left superior lobar bronchus

Left inferior lobar bronchus

Right and left atria

Left lung, inferior lobe

PLATE **47b** THORACIC ORGANS, INTERMEDIATE VIEW—MODEL

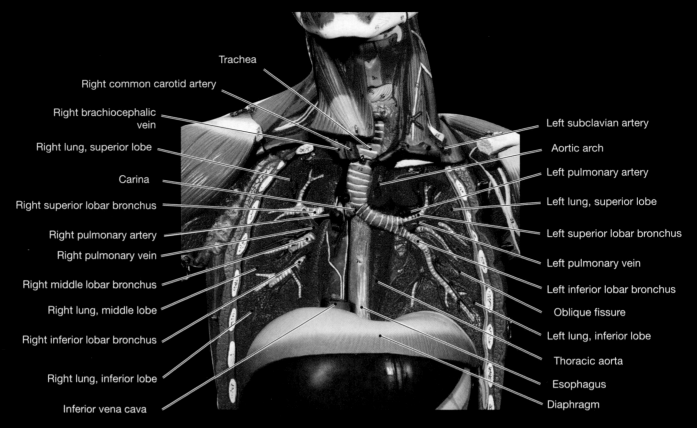

Trachea

Right common carotid artery

Right brachiocephalic vein

Right lung, superior lobe

Carina

Right superior lobar bronchus

Right pulmonary artery

Right pulmonary vein

Right middle lobar bronchus

Right lung, middle lobe

Right inferior lobar bronchus

Right lung, inferior lobe

Inferior vena cava

Left subclavian artery

Aortic arch

Left pulmonary artery

Left lung, superior lobe

Left superior lobar bronchus

Left pulmonary vein

Left inferior lobar bronchus

Oblique fissure

Left lung, inferior lobe

Thoracic aorta

Esophagus

Diaphragm

PLATE 47c THORACIC ORGANS, DEEPER VIEW—MODEL

Internal thoracic vein

Carina

Azygos vein

Intercostal vein, artery, and nerve

Parietal pleura (right lung removed)

Esophagus

Inferior vena cava

Diaphragm

Right kidney

Left common carotid artery

Thyrocervical trunk

Brachial plexus

Left axillary artery

Left external jugular vein

Left internal jugular vein

Left subclavian vein

Left brachiocephalic vein

Thoracic aorta

Visceral pleura covering base of left lung

Abdominal aorta

Left kidney

PLATE 47d THE THORACIC CAVITY

PLATE **48b** LYMPHANGIOGRAM OF THORAX,
ANTERIOR–POSTERIOR PROJECTION

Lymph
nodes

Apex of
heart

Diaphragm

Descending
colon

Transverse
colon

Left lateral
aortic lymph
node

Right lumbar
trunk

Left lumbar
trunk

Iliac crest

Descending
colon

External iliac
lymph nodes

Superficial
inguinal
lymph nodes

Thoracic
aorta

Thoracic duct

Diaphragm

First lumbar
vertebra

Cisterna chyli

Abdominal
aorta

PLATE **48a** LYMPHATIC TRUNK

PLATE **48c** LYMPHANGIOGRAM OF PELVIS, ANTERIOR PROJECTION

Esophagus

Diaphragm

Right lobe
of liver

Gallbladder

Transverse
colon

Ascending
colon

Cecum

Appendix

Falciform
ligament
of liver

Left lobe
of liver

Stomach

Greater omentum
(cut)

Tenia coli

Jejunum } Small
Ileum } intestine

Sigmoid
colon

PLATE 49a THE ABDOMINOPELVIC VISCERA, SUPERFICIAL ANTERIOR VIEW

Inferior lobe of right lung

Falciform ligament

Diaphragm

eft lobe of liver

Right lobe of liver

Gallbladder

Transverse colon

Pericardium

Inferior lobe of left lung

Stomach

Greater omentum

PLATE 49b SUPERIOR PORTION OF ABDOMINOPELVIC CAVITY, ANTERIOR VIEW

Liver (right lobe)

Falciform ligament

Gallbladder

Transverse colon

Fatty appendices of colon

Ascending colon

Stomach

Liver (left lobe)

Greater omentum

PLATE 49c INFERIOR PORTION OF ABDOMINOPELVIC CAVITY, ANTERIOR VIEW

Liver
(left and
right lobes)

Gallbladder

Transverse
colon

Jejunum

Ascending
colon

Ileum

Cecum

Greater
omentum
(reflected)

Transverse
colon

Fatty
appendices
of colon

Descending
colon

PLATE **49d** ABDOMINAL DISSECTION, GREATER OMENTUM REFLECTED

Falciform ligament

Cystic duct

Right lobe
of liver

Gallbladder

Common bile duct

Duodenum

Pylorus

Pancreas

Right kidney

Inferior vena cava

Aorta

Diaphragm

Left lobe
of liver

Left gastric
artery

Spleen

Stomach

Left kidney

Greater
omentum

Cauda equina

PLATE **49e** LIVER AND GALLBLADDER IN SITU

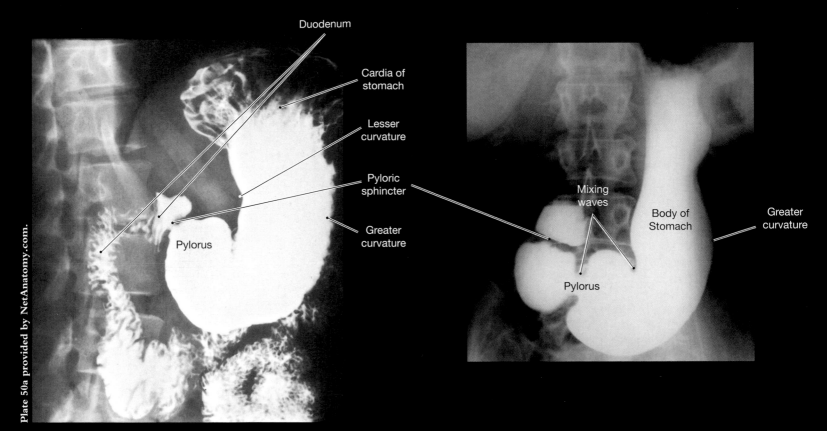

Duodenum

Cardia of stomach

Lesser curvature

Pyloric sphincter

Greater curvature

Pylorus

Plate 50a provided by NetAnatomy.com.

PLATE **50a** GASTRIC RADIOGRAM 1

Mixing waves

Body of Stomach

Greater curvature

Pylorus

PLATE **50b** GASTRIC RADIOGRAM 2

Pylorus

Mixing wave, time 1

Body of stomach

Pylorus

Body of stomach

Mixing waves, time 2

PLATE **50c** GASTRIC MOTILITY, ANTERIOR VIEW, TIMES 1 AND 2

Right lobe of liver

Hepatic artery

Bile duct

Common hepatic artery

Splenic artery

Gastroduodenal artery

Gallbladder

Probe in duodenal ampulla

Duodenum

Transverse colon

Stomach

Plicae circulares (circular folds)

PLATE 51a ABDOMINAL DISSECTION, DUODENAL REGION

PLATE 51b GROSS ANATOMY OF DUODENAL MUCOSA

Probe in duodenal ampulla

Plicae circulares (circular folds)

Plicae circulares (circular folds)

Jejunum

PLATE 51c GROSS ANATOMY OF THE JEJUNAL MUCOSA

Plicae circulares (circular folds)

Ileum

PLATE 51d GROSS ANATOMY OF THE ILEAL MUCOSA

Polyp
on wall
of colon

Normal section
of colon,
after removal
of a polyp

PLATE 52 ABNORMAL AND NORMAL COLONOSCOPE

Right lobe
of liver

Transverse
colon

Middle colic
artery

Superior
mesenteric
artery

Ascending
colon

Ileocolic artery

Jejunal
arteries

Cecum

Jejunum

Descending
colon

PLATE 53a BRANCHES OF THE SUPERIOR MESENTERIC ARTERY

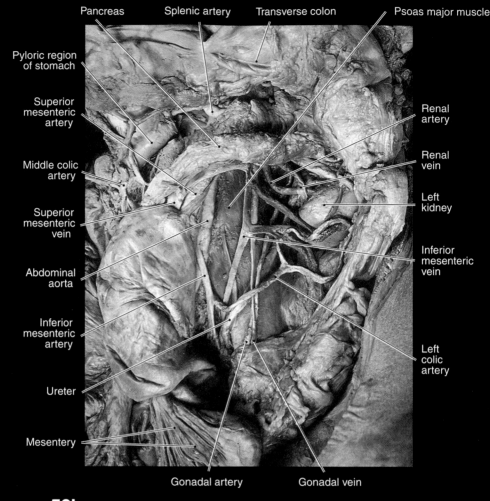

Pancreas Splenic artery Transverse colon Psoas major muscle

Pyloric region
of stomach

Superior
mesenteric
artery

Middle colic
artery

Superior
mesenteric
vein

Abdominal
aorta

Inferior
mesenteric
artery

Ureter

Mesentery

Renal
artery

Renal
vein

Left
kidney

Inferior
mesenteric
vein

Left
colic
artery

Gonadal artery Gonadal vein

PLATE **53b** INFERIOR MESENTERIC VESSELS

Celiac trunk

Right renal
artery

Superior
mesenteric
artery

Internal
iliac artery

Abdominal
aorta

Left renal
artery

Lumbar
artery

Common
iliac artery

External
iliac artery

PLATE **53c** ABDOMINAL ARTERIOGRAM 1

PLATE **53d** ABDOMINAL ARTERIOGRAM 2

Cystic artery

Hepatic artery

Common hepatic artery

Gastroduodenal artery

Right adrenal artery

Right renal artery

Superior mesenteric artery

Right kidney

Splenic artery

Celiac trunk

Left adrenal artery

Left renal artery

Left kidney

Common hepatic artery

Celiac trunk

Pancreaticoduodenal artery

Right colic artery

Ileocolic artery

Common iliac artery

Left gastric artery

Splenic artery

Superior mesenteric artery

Left renal artery

Intestinal arteries

Terminal segment of the aorta

PLATE **53e** ABDOMINAL ARTERIOGRAM 3 (COLORIZED)

Coronary ligament

Posterior

Inferior
vena cava

Diaphragm

Parietal
pericardium

Right

Left

Right lobe

Left lobe

Falciform
ligament

Anterior

PLATE **54a** THE ISOLATED LIVER AND GALLBLADDER, SUPERIOR VIEW

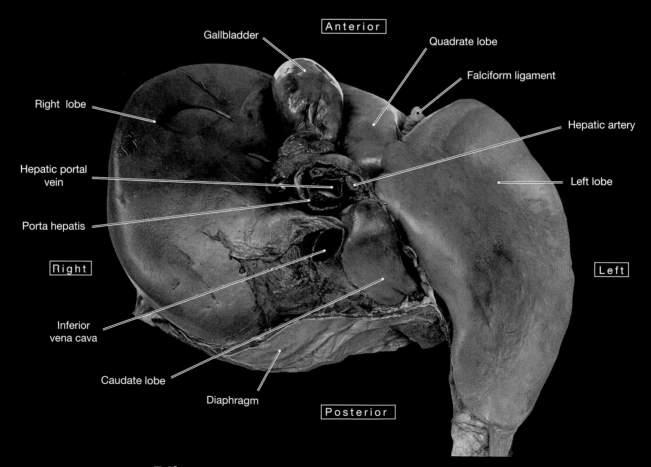

Anterior

Gallbladder

Quadrate lobe

Falciform ligament

Right lobe

Hepatic artery

Hepatic portal
vein

Left lobe

Porta hepatis

Right

Left

Inferior
vena cava

Caudate lobe

Diaphragm

Posterior

PLATE **54b** THE ISOLATED LIVER AND GALLBLADDER, INFERIOR VIEW

PLATE **54c** CORROSION
CAST OF LIVER

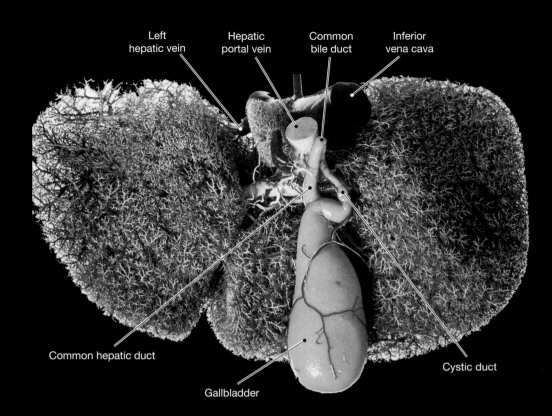

Left
hepatic vein

Hepatic
portal vein

Common
bile duct

Inferior
vena cava

Common hepatic duct

Cystic duct

Gallbladder

Left hepatic duct

Right
hepatic duct

Gallbladder

Cystic
duct

Common
bile duct

Duodenum

PLATE **54d** CHOLANGIOPANCREATOGRAM (PANCREATIC
AND BILE DUCTS)

Splenic vein

Pancreatic
duct

Pancreatic
vein

Splenic artery

Pancreatic arteries

PLATE **55** CORROSION CAST OF SPLENIC AND PANCREATIC
VESSELS

Head of humerus

Coracoid process of scapula

Clavicle

First rib

Trachea

Vertebral body (T₁)

Spinal cord

Transverse process

Spinous process

R

L

56a

Sternum

Lungs

Vertebral body

Spinal cord

Ribs

Heart

Aorta

56b

PLATES **56a–b** MRI SCANS OF THE TRUNK, HORIZONTAL SECTIONS, SUPERIOR TO INFERIOR SEQUENCE

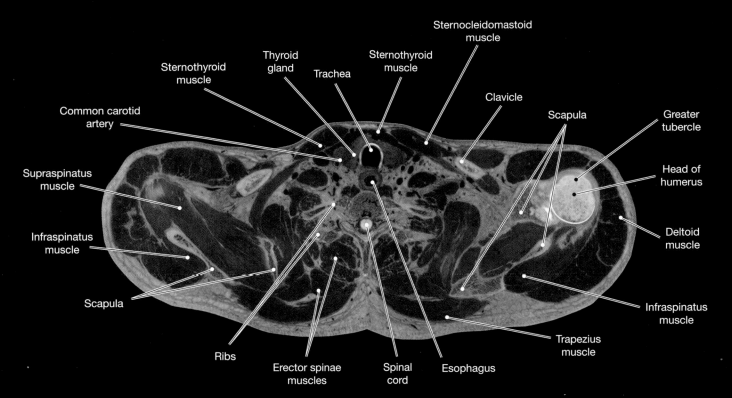

Sternocleidomastoid
muscle

Thyroid
gland

Sternothyroid
muscle

Sternothyroid
muscle

Trachea

Clavicle

Scapula

Greater
tubercle

Common carotid
artery

Head of
humerus

Supraspinatus
muscle

Deltoid
muscle

Infraspinatus
muscle

Scapula

Infraspinatus
muscle

Trapezius
muscle

Ribs

Erector spinae
muscles

Spinal
cord

Esophagus

56c

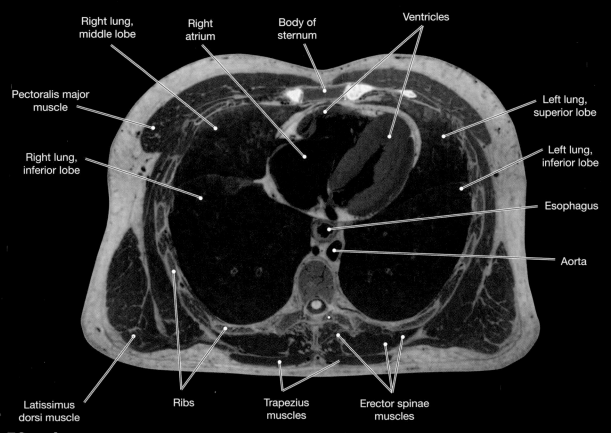

Right lung,
middle lobe

Right
atrium

Body of
sternum

Ventricles

Pectoralis major
muscle

Left lung,
superior lobe

Right lung,
inferior lobe

Left lung,
inferior lobe

Esophagus

Aorta

Latissimus
dorsi muscle

Ribs

Trapezius
muscles

Erector spinae
muscles

56d

PLATES 56c–d HORIZONTAL SECTIONS THROUGH THE TRUNK

These sections, derived from the Visible Human dataset, are at the approximate levels of the scans shown in parts a–b.

Diaphragm

Transverse colon

Stomach

Liver

Aorta

Pleural cavity

Spleen

Diaphragm

Erector spinae muscles

56e

Hepatic portal vein

Inferior vena cava

Liver, left lobe

Stomach

Liver, right lobe

Transverse colon

Ribs

Latissimus dorsi muscle

Diaphragm

Erector spinae

PLATES 56e–f HORIZONTAL SECTIONS THROUGH THE TRUNK

Section f, derived from the Visible Human dataset, is at the approximate level of the scan shown in part e.

56f

Hepatic portal vein

Falciform ligament

Abdominal aorta

Superior mesenteric artery

Inferior vena cava

Left lobe

Stomach

Hepatic duct

Splenic vein

Diaphgragm

Right lobe

Spleen

Liver

Transverse colon

12th rib

Descending colon

Pancreas

Left kidney

Right kidney

Inferior tip of spinal cord

Erector spinae muscle group

Quadratus lumborum muscle

PLATE 57a ABDOMINAL CAVITY, HORIZONTAL SECTION AT T_{12}

Falciform ligament

Left lobe of liver

Cut edge of diaphragm

Parietal peritoneum

Pleural cavity

Caudate lobe of liver

Stomach

Inferior vena cava

Aorta

Right lobe of liver

Spleen

Left kidney

PLATE 57b ABDOMINAL CAVITY, HORIZONTAL SECTION AT L_1

Transverse colon

Superior mesenteric artery

Small intestine

Superior mesenteric vein

Colon

Liver

Renal vein

Pancreas

Aorta

Inferior vena cava

Renal artery

Renal pelvis

Right kidney

Left kidney

Erector spinae muscles

58a

Ileum

Jejunum

Ascending colon

Descending colon

Inferior vena cava

Abdominal aorta

Transverse process of third lumbar vertebra

Iliopsoas muscle

Cauda equina

Spinous process of third lumbar vertebra

Longissimus muscle

58b

PLATES 58a–b MRI SCANS OF THE TRUNK, HORIZONTAL SECTIONS, SUPERIOR TO INFERIOR SEQUENCE

Transverse colon

Rectus abdominis muscle

Aorta

Small intestine

Ascending colon

Descending colon

Liver

Renal vein

Right kidney

Vertebra L₁

Ureter

Left kidney

Renal artery

Quadratus lumborum muscle

Spinalis thoracis muscle

Longissimus thoracis muscle

Psoas major muscle

Iliocostalis lumborum muscle

58c

Ascending colon

Inferior vena cava

Aorta

Rectus abdominis muscle

Small intestine

External oblique muscle

Internal oblique muscle

Descending colon

Transversus abdominis muscle

Psoas major muscle

Quadratus lumborum muscle

Erector spinae muscles

Cauda equina

58d

PLATES **58c–d**
HORIZONTAL SECTIONS
THROUGH THE TRUNK

These sections, derived from the Visible Human dataset, are at the approximate levels of the scans shown in parts a–b.

Descending colon

Cecum

Iliacus muscle

Urinary bladder

Psoas major muscle

Ureters

Gluteus minimus muscle

Sigmoid colon

Ilia

Gluteus medius muscle

Sacrum

Gluteus maximus muscle

58e

Rectus abdominis muscle

Iliacus muscle

Gluteus minimus muscle

Psoas major muscle

Ilium

Gluteus medius muscle

Gluteus maximus muscle

Sacrum

Sacroiliac joint

Common iliac vein

Common iliac artery

58f

PLATES 58e–f HORIZONTAL SECTIONS THROUGH THE TRUNK

Part f, derived from the Visible Human dataset, is at the approximate level of the MRI scan in part e.

Right colic
(hepatic) flexure

Left colic
(splenic) flexure

Haustra

Transverse colon

Ascending colon

Descending colon

Cecum

Sigmoid colon

Rectum

PLATE **59** CONTRAST X-RAY OF COLON AND RECTUM, ANTERIOR-POSTERIOR PROJECTION

PLATE 60a Testis and epididymis

Spermatic cord

Ductus deferens

Head of epididymis

Body of epididymis

Tunica albuginea covering testis

Tunica vaginalis (reflected)

Tail of epididymis

PLATE 60b Cross section through dissected penis

Pubic symphysis

Dorsal artery

Superficial dorsal vein

Deep dorsal vein

Dorsal artery

Corpora cavernosa

Spongy urethra

Corpus spongiosum

Ischiocavernosus muscle

Bulbospongiosus muscle overlying shaft of penis

Hepatic vein (stump)

Left renal vein

Right adrenal gland

Inferior vena cava

Right renal vein

Right renal artery

Right kidney

Peritoneum

Right ureter

Right gonadal vein

Inferior mesenteric artery

Left gastric artery

Common hepatic artery

Splenic artery

Celiac trunk

Celiac ganglion

Left adrenal gland

Left adrenal vein

Left renal vein

Left renal artery

Left kidney

Superior mesenteric artery

Left ureter

Left gonadal vein

Gonadal arteries

Abdominal aorta

PLATE 61a The posterior abdominal wall

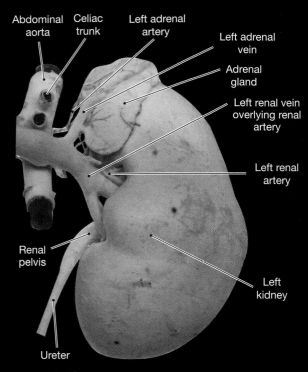

Abdominal aorta
Celiac trunk
Left adrenal artery
Left adrenal vein
Adrenal gland
Left renal vein overlying renal artery
Left renal artery
Renal pelvis
Left kidney
Ureter

PLATE 61b LEFT KIDNEY, ANTERIOR VIEW

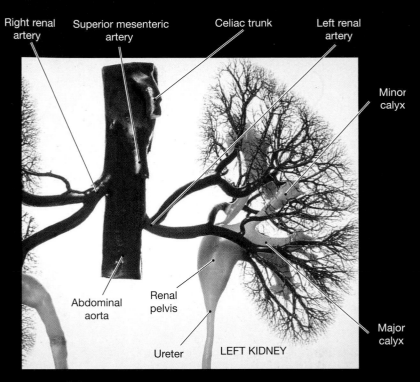

Right renal artery
Superior mesenteric artery
Celiac trunk
Left renal artery
Minor calyx
Abdominal aorta
Renal pelvis
Ureter
LEFT KIDNEY
Major calyx

PLATE 61c CORROSION CAST OF THE RENAL ARTERIES, URETERS, AND RENAL PELVIS

Diaphragm
Right lobe of liver (cut)
Right adrenal gland
Right kidney
Inferior vena cava
Quadratus lumborum muscle
Right ureter
Psoas major muscle
Iliacus muscle

Spleen
Left middle adrenal vein
Left renal artery
Left kidney
Left renal vein
Superior mesenteric artery
Inferior mesenteric artery
Abdominal aorta
Left common iliac artery and vein
Left internal iliac artery
Left external iliac artery
Left external iliac vein

PLATE 62a THE ABDOMINOPELVIC CAVITY, FEMALE, ANTERIOR VIEW—MODEL

Right kidney

Adrenal artery
and vein

Transversus
abdominis
muscle

Inferior vena cava

Abdominal aorta

Quadratus
lumborum
muscle

Psoas major
muscle

Iliacus muscle

Anterior superior
iliac spine

Urinary bladder

Prostate gland

Adrenal gland

Phrenic artery
and vein

Celiac trunk

Left kidney

Renal artery

Renal vein

Superior mesenteric
artery

Ureter

Lumbar artery

Testicular
artery and vein

Inferior
mesenteric
artery

Common
iliac artery

Common
iliac vein

Rectum

Prostatic urethra

Pubic symphysis

PLATE **62b** THE ABDOMINOPELVIC CAVITY, MALE, ANTERIOR VIEW—MODEL

Internal
oblique muscle

Iliohypogastric
nerve

Ilioinguinal
nerve

Deep inguinal
ring

Aponeurosis of
(reflected) external
oblique muscle

Inguinal canal

Scrotal branch of
ilioinguinal nerve

Rectus abdominis
muscle

Cremasteric muscle
and fascia
surrounding
spermatic cord

Edge of superficial
inguinal ring

Ductus deferens

PLATE **63** RIGHT LOWER
QUADRANT (RLQ), MALE

Sigmoid colon

Rectus abdominis muscle

Urinary bladder

Pubic symphysis

Spongy urethra within corpus spongiosum

Penis

Corpus cavernosum

Epididymis

Testis

Rectum

Internal urethral orifice

Prostatic urethra

Prostate gland

Ejaculatory duct

Membranous urethra

Penile urethra

Bulbospongiosus muscle

Ductus deferens

Scrotum

PLATE 64 PELVIC REGION OF A MALE, SAGITTAL SECTION

Sigmoid colon (cut and reflected)

Urinary bladder

Pubic symphysis

Urethra

External urethral orifice

Vestibule

Fat of mons pubis

Labium minus

Labium majus

Suspensory ligament of ovary

Uterine tube

Ovary

Fundus of uterus

Endometrium of uterus

Body of uterus (myometrium)

Probe through internal os

Cervix

Probe through cervical os

Vagina

Rectum

Anus

PLATE 65 PELVIC REGION OF A FEMALE, SAGITTAL SECTION

Ovarian ligament

POSTERIOR

Infundibulum

Ovary

Suspensory ligament

Uterine tube

Ampulla

Ovarian hilum

Mesovarium

Isthmus

Round ligament

Fundus of uterus

Posterior surface of broad ligament

Urinary bladder

ANTERIOR

PLATE 66 PELVIC CAVITY, SUPERIOR VIEW

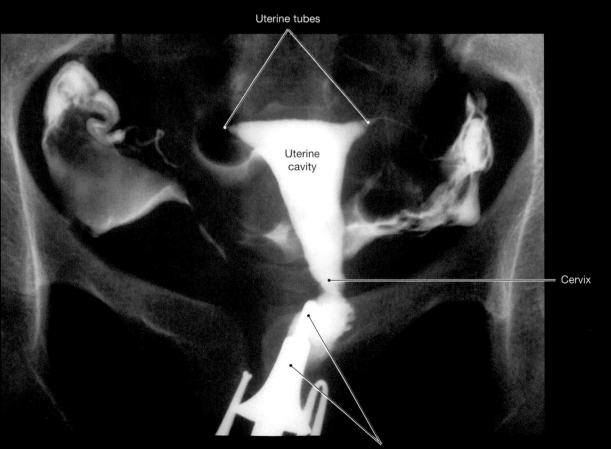

Uterine tubes

Uterine cavity

Cervix

Application tube in vagina, source of contrast medium

PLATE 67 HYSTEROSALPINGOGRAM

Iliac crest

Posterior superior Iliac spine

Greater trochanter of femur

Location of sciatic nerve

Hamstring muscle group

Tendon of biceps femoris muscle

Tendon of semitendinosus muscle

Median sacral crest

Gluteal injection site

Gluteus medius muscle

Gluteus maximus muscle

Fold of buttock

Popliteal fossa

Site for palpation of popliteal artery

Lumbodorsal (thoracolumbar) fascia

Cutaneous branches of L_1–L_3

Gluteus maximus muscle

Levator ani muscle

Adductor magnus muscle

Gracilis muscle

Semitendinosus muscle

PLATE 68b SUPERFICIAL DISSECTION OF THE RIGHT HIP, POSTERIOR VIEW

PLATE 68a GLUTEAL REGION AND THIGHS

Superior gluteal artery

Lateral sacral artery

Ventral rami of S_1-S_3

Piriformis muscle

Inferior gluteal artery

Coccygeus muscle

Internal pudendal artery

Obturator internus muscle

Sacral promontory

Internal iliac artery

External iliac artery

Obturator artery

Inferior epigastric artery

Pubic symphysis

PLATE 68c BLOOD VESSELS, NERVES, AND MUSCLES IN THE LEFT HALF OF THE PELVIS

Tensor fasciae
latae muscle

Gluteus
medius muscle

Gluteus
maximus muscle

Iliotibial tract

Vastus lateralis

Semitendinosus and
semimembranosus
muscles

Tendon of biceps
femoris muscle

Popliteal fossa

Patella

Patellar ligament

Tibial tuberosity

Head of fibula

Gastrocnemius
muscle

Soleus
muscle

Fibularis
longus muscle

PLATE **69a** SURFACE ANATOMY OF THE THIGH,
LATERAL VIEW

Tensor
fasciae
latae
muscle

Sartorius
muscle

Rectus
femoris
muscle

Vastus
lateralis
muscle

Vastus
medialis
muscle

Patella

Tibial
tuberosity

Inguinal
ligament

Area of
femoral
triangle, site
for palpation
of femoral
artery

Adductor
longus
muscle

Gracilis
muscle

PLATE **69b** SURFACE ANATOMY OF RIGHT THIGH,
ANTERIOR VIEW

Inguinal ligament

Femoral artery

Deep inguinal lymph nodes

Great saphenous vein

Inguinal ligament

Iliopsoas muscle

Sartorius muscle

Fascia overlying tensor fasciae latae

Lateral circumflex artery

Rectus femoris muscle

Femoral artery

Femoral nerve

Femoral vein

Pectineus muscle

Great saphenous vein

Adductor brevis muscle

Adductor longus muscle

Deep femoral artery

Saphenous nerve overlying femoral artery

PLATE 70a DISSECTION OF THE RIGHT INGUINAL REGION, MALE

PLATE 70b SUPERFICIAL DISSECTION OF THE RIGHT THIGH, ANTERIOR VIEW

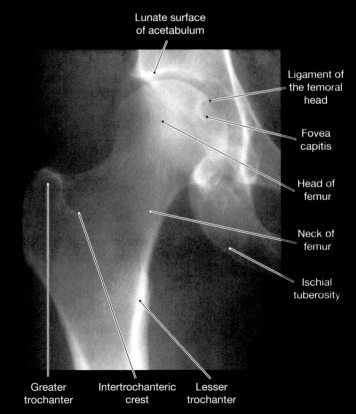

Lunate surface of acetabulum

Vertebra L₅

Left ala of sacrum

Left sacroiliac joint

Anterior superior iliac spine

Sacral foramina

Lesser trochanter of right femur

Pelvic inlet

Ischium

Pubis

Pubic tubercle

Pubic symphsis

Obturator foramen

Arcuate line

Greater trochanter of left femur

Lunate surface of acetabulum

Ligament of the femoral head

Fovea capitis

Head of femur

Neck of femur

Ischial tuberosity

Greater trochanter

Intertrochanteric crest

Lesser trochanter

PLATE 71a X-RAY OF PELVIS AND PROXIMAL FEMORA, ANTERIOR–POSTERIOR PROJECTION

PLATE 71b X-RAY OF THE RIGHT HIP JOINT, ANTERIOR–POSTERIOR PROJECTION

External
iliac
artery

Psoas
major muscle

Iliac crest

Iliacus muscle

Gluteus medius
muscle

Gluteus minimus
muscle

Fibrocartilage
of lunate
surface

Acetabular
labrum

Articular cartilage
of femoral head

Head of femur

Greater trochanter

Neck of femur

Articular capsule

Iliacus muscle

Pectineus muscle

Vastus lateralis muscle

Adductor longus muscle

Vastus medialis muscle

PLATE 72a CORONAL SECTION THROUGH THE LEFT HIP

Psoas major muscle

Iliac crest

Iliacus muscle

Gluteus medius muscle

Gluteus minimus muscle

Superior lip of acetabulum

Head of femur

Piriformis muscle

Greater trochanter

Obturator internus muscle

Obturator externus muscle

Ischium

Adductor brevis muscle

Vastus lateralis muscle

Adductor magnus muscle

Gracilis muscle

Deep femoral artery

Vastus intermedius muscle

Sacrum

External iliac arteries

Vastus intermedius muscle

PLATE 72b MRI SCAN OF PELVIC REGION, FRONTAL SECTION

Iliac crest

Iliacus muscle

Anterior superior
iliac spine

Inguinal ligament

Sartorius muscle

Tensor fasciae
latae muscle

Vastus lateralis
muscle

Rectus femoris
muscle

Psoas major muscle

Piriformis muscle

Coccygeus muscle

Pectineus muscle

Pubic tubercle

Adductor brevis muscle

Adductor longus muscle

Gracilis muscle

L₅

Sacral canal

Piriformis
muscle

Coccygeus
muscle

Coccyx

Gluteus
maximus
muscle

Adductor
magnus
muscle

Psoas major
muscle

Iliacus
muscle

Anterior
iliac spine

Pubococcygeus
muscle
(levator ani)

Obturator
internus
muscle

Pubic
symphysis

Adductor
longus
muscle

Gracilis
muscle

Iliac crest

Inguinal ligament

Tensor fasciae latae muscle

Great saphenous vein

Rectus femoris muscle

Vastus lateralis muscle

Iliopsoas muscle

Femoral nerve

Sartorius muscle

Femoral artery

Adductor brevis muscle

Adductor longus muscle

Gracilis muscle

Vastus medialis

Quadriceps tendon

Patella

Patellar ligament

PLATE 74 SUPERFICIAL DISSECTION OF RIGHT LOWER LIMB, ANTERIOR VIEW

Articular surface of head

Neck

Greater trochanter

Intertrochanteric line

Lesser trochanter

Shaft of femur

Medial epicondyle

Patellar surface

Lateral epicondyle

Lateral condyle

Medial condyle

PLATE 75a RIGHT FEMUR, ANTERIOR VIEW

Femoral head

Neck

Greater trochanter

Lesser trochanter

Adductor tubercle

Lateral condyle

Medial condyle

PLATE 75b RIGHT FEMUR, SUPERIOR VIEW

Greater trochanter

Intertrochanteric line

Neck

Articular surface of head

PLATE 75c HEAD OF RIGHT FEMUR, LATERAL VIEW

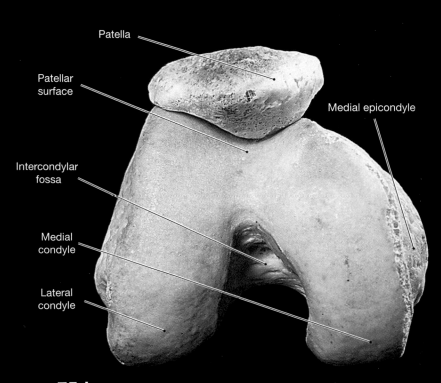

Patella

Patellar surface

Medial epicondyle

Intercondylar fossa

Medial condyle

Lateral condyle

PLATE 75d RIGHT FEMUR, INFERIOR VIEW

Gluteus maximus
muscle

Adductor magnus
muscle

Vastus lateralis muscle
covered by iliotibial tract

Semitendinosus
muscle

Biceps femoris
muscle, long head

⎫
⎬ Hamstrings
⎭

Semimembranosus
muscle

Tendon of
biceps femoris,
short head

Popliteal fossa

Medial head of
gastrocnemius muscle

Lateral head of
gastrocnemius muscle

PLATE **76a** SURFACE ANATOMY OF RIGHT THIGH,
POSTERIOR VIEW

Iliac crest

Gluteal aponeurosis
over gluteus medius
muscle

Gluteus maximus
muscle

Tensor fasciae
latae muscle

Sciatic nerve

Iliotibial tract
over vastus
lateralis muscle

Adductor
magnus
muscle

Biceps femoris
muscle, long head

Semitendinosus
muscle

Biceps femoris
muscle, short head

Gracilis
muscle

Semimembranosus
muscle

Popliteal
vein

Semitendinosus
muscle

Tibial nerve

Tendon of
gracilis

Sartorius
muscle

Medial head
of gastrocnemius
muscle

Lateral head
of gastrocnemius
muscle

Articular
surface
of head

Neck

Greater
trochanter

Intertrochanteric
crest

Gluteal
tuberosity

Lesser
trochanter

Pectineal
line

Linea
aspera

Lateral
supracondylar
ridge

Medial
supracondylar
ridge

Popliteal
surface

Adductor
tubercle

Medial
epicondyle

Lateral
epicondyle

Lateral
condyle

Medial
condyle

Intercondylar
fossa

Semimembranosus
muscle

Semitendinosus
muscle

Tibial nerve

Femur

Popliteus
muscle

Gastrocnemius
muscle

Soleus
muscle

Popliteal artery (red)
and vein (blue)

Tendon of
quadriceps
muscles

Suprapatellar
bursa

Articular
cartilage
of patella

Patella

Articular
cartilage of femur
(patellar surface)

Patellar fat pad

Patellar ligament

Lateral meniscus

Anterior
cruciate ligament

Posterior
cruciate ligament

Tibia

PLATE 78a THE KNEE, PARASAGITTAL SECTION—MODEL

PLATE 77 RIGHT FEMUR, POSTERIOR VIEW

78b

Patellar surface

Patella

Intercondylar fossa

Posterior cruciate ligament

Lateral condyle

Medial condyle

Anterior cruciate ligament

Sartorius muscle

Great saphenous vein

Biceps femoris muscle

Tendon of gracilis muscle

Tendon of semimembranosus muscle

Popliteal artery

Popliteal vein

Tibial nerve

Tendon of semitendinosus muscle

Patellar ligament

Tibia

Popliteus muscle

Sartorius muscle

Head of fibula

Great saphenous vein

Tendon of semitendinosus muscle

Gastrocnemius muscle, lateral head

Gastrocnemius muscle, medial head

PLATES **78b–c** MRI SCANS OF THE RIGHT KNEE, HORIZONTAL SECTIONS, SUPERIOR TO INFERIOR SEQUENCE

78c

78d

Patella

Quadriceps tendon

Fat body (prefemoral)

Semimembranosus muscle

Popliteal vein

Articular cartilage of femur

Femur

Infrapatellar fat pad

Gastrocnemius muscle, lateral head

Patellar ligament

Articular cartilage of tibia

Lateral meniscus

Tibia

Popliteus muscle

Tibial tuberosity

Soleus muscle

Patella

Quadriceps tendon

Cartilage of patella

Deep popliteal vein

Semimembranosus muscle

Popliteal vein

Joint capsule

Femur

Popliteal artery

Gastrocnemius muscle, lateral head

Patellar ligament

Tibia

Popliteus muscle

Soleus muscle

PLATES 78d–e MRI SCANS OF THE RIGHT KNEE, PARASAGITTAL SECTIONS, LATERAL TO MEDIAL SEQUENCE

78e

78f

Iliotibial tract

Deep popliteal vein

Popliteal vein

Semimembranosus muscle

Sartorius muscle

11-JUL-94
5:17:54

Biceps femoris muscle

Lateral condyle

Popliteus muscle

Head of fibula

Gastrocnemius muscle, lateral head

Medial condyle

Gracilis muscle

Tibia

Posterior edge of joint capsule

Gastrocnemius muscle, medial head

g f

PLATES 78f–g MRI SCANS OF THE RIGHT KNEE, FRONTAL SECTIONS, POSTERIOR TO ANTERIOR SEQUENCE

78g

Biceps femoris muscle

Popliteal vein

Intercondylar fossa

Vastus medialis muscle

Posterior cruciate ligament

11-JUL-94
13:17:54

Anterior cruciate ligament

Lateral condyle of femur

Fibular collateral ligament

Lateral meniscus

Tubercles of intercondylar eminence of tibia

Epiphyseal line

Tibia

Medial condyle of femur

Medial meniscus

Tibial collateral ligament

Great saphenous vein

Gastrocnemius muscle, medial head

Lateral
epicondyle

FEMUR

Patella

Medial
epicondyle

Femoral
epicondyle

Intercondylar
eminence

Lateral
tibial
condyle

Medial
tibial
condyle

Head of
fibula

TIBIA

Shaft of
fibula

PLATE **78h** X-RAY OF THE EXTENDED RIGHT KNEE, ANTERIOR-POSTERIOR PROJECTION

Femoral
condyle

FEMUR

Quadriceps
muscles

Quadriceps
tendon

Intercondylar
eminence
of tibia

Patella

Medial
tibial
condyle

Patellar
ligamant

FIBULA

Tibial
tuberosity

TIBIA

PLATE **78i** X-RAY OF THE PARTIALLY FLEXED RIGHT KNEE, LATERAL PROJECTION

Anterior cruciate ligament

Femur

Medial condyle

Fibular collateral ligament

Tibial collateral ligament

Lateral condyle

Lateral meniscus

Medial meniscus

Posterior cruciate ligament

Cut tendon of biceps femoris muscle

Tibia

Head of fibula

PLATE 79a EXTENDED RIGHT KNEE, POSTERIOR VIEW

Articular cartilage

Patellar surface

Lateral condyle

Medial condyle

Fibular collateral ligament

Posterior cruciate ligament

Lateral meniscus

Tibial collateral ligament

Cut tendon of biceps femoris muscle

Medial meniscus

Anterior cruciate ligament

Fibula

Tibia

PLATE 79b EXTENDED RIGHT KNEE, ANTERIOR VIEW

Articular surface of medial condyle

Tibial tuberosity

Articular surface of lateral condyle

Tubercles of intercondylar eminence

PLATE 80a PROXIMAL END OF RIGHT TIBIA, SUPERIOR VIEW

Lateral malleolus (fibula)

Inferior articular surface for ankle joint

Medial malleolus (tibia)

PLATE 80b DISTAL END OF TIBIA AND FIBULA, INFERIOR VIEW

Rectus femoris
muscle

Vastus medialis
muscle

Vastus lateralis
muscle

Patella

Tibial tuberosity

Fibularis longus
muscle

Gastrocnemius
muscle

Anterior border
of tibia

Soleus muscle

Tibialis anterior
muscle

Great saphenous
vein

Medial malleolus

Lateral malleolus

Dorsal venous
arch

Tendon of extensor
hallucis longus

Tendons of extensor
digitorum longus

PLATE 81a SURFACE ANATOMY OF
THE RIGHT LEG AND FOOT, ANTERIOR
VIEW

Vastus lateralis
muscle

Vastus medialis
muscle

Quadriceps
tendon

Patella

Medial
condyle
of femur

Patellar
ligament

Gastrocnemius
muscle

Tibialis anterior
muscle

Soleus muscle

Tibia

Extensor digitorum
longus muscle

Extensor hallucis
longus muscle

Medial malleolus

Lateral malleolus

PLATE 81b SUPERFICIAL
DISSECTION OF THE RIGHT LEG AND
FOOT, ANTERIOR VIEW

Site for palpation of popliteal artery

Site for palpation of common peroneal nerve

Gastrocnemius muscle, lateral head

Gastrocnemius muscle, medial head

Soleus muscle

Calcaneal tendon

Medial malleolus

Site for palpation of posterior tibial artery

Tendon of fibularis longus

Lateral malleolus

Calcaneus

PLATE **82a** SURFACE ANATOMY OF THE RIGHT LEG AND FOOT, POSTERIOR VIEW

Tendon of gracilis

Tendon of semitendinosus

Tendon of semimembranosus

Gastrocnemius muscle, medial head

Plantaris muscle (cut)

Gastrocnemius muscle, lateral head

Tibial nerve

Tendon of biceps femoris

Common fibular nerve

Plantaris muscle (cut)

Soleus muscle

Fibularis longus muscle

Tendon of tibialis posterior

Calcaneal tendon

Flexor hallucis longus muscle

Flexor digitorum longus muscle

Fibularis brevis muscle

PLATE **82b** SUPERFICIAL DISSECTION OF THE RIGHT LEG AND FOOT, POSTERIOR VIEW

Lateral condyle of tibia

Medial condyle of tibia

Head of fibula

Superior tibiofibular joint

Tibial tuberosity

Interosseous border of fibula

Anterior margin

Shaft of fibula

Interosseous border of tibia

Shaft of tibia

Inferior tibiofibular joint

Medial malleolus

Lateral malleolus

Inferior articular surface

PLATE 83a TIBIA AND FIBULA, ANTERIOR VIEW

Medial tubercle of intercondylar eminence

Lateral tubercle of intercondylar eminence

Articular surface of medial condyle

Intercondylar eminence

Medial condyle

Lateral condyle

Head of fibula

Popliteal line

TIBIA

FIBULA

Medial malleolus

Articular surfaces of tibia and fibula

Lateral malleolus

PLATE 83b TIBIA AND FIBULA, POSTERIOR VIEW

Vastus
lateralis
muscle

Biceps femoris
muscle,
short head

Iliotibial
tract

Patella

Lateral head
of
gastrocnemius
muscle

Head of
fibula

Patellar
ligament

Tibialis anterior
muscle

Soleus
muscle

Fibularis longus
muscle

Superficial
fibular nerve

Calcaneal
tendon

Fibularis brevis
muscle

Calcaneus

Extensor digitorum
longus muscle

Lateral malleolus

Inferior extensor
retinaculum

PLATE **84a** SUPERFICIAL DISSECTION OF THE
RIGHT LEG AND FOOT, ANTEROLATERAL VIEW

Sural nerve

Fibularis brevis
muscle

Fibularis longus
muscle

Extensor digitorum
longus muscle

Soleus muscle

Fibula

Flexor hallucis
longus muscle

Superior extensor
retinaculum

Calcaneal
tendon

Inferior extensor
retinaculum

Tendon of
fibularis longus

Tendons of
extensor digitorum
longus muscle

Calcaneus

Extensor hallucis
longus muscle

Tendon of
fibularis brevis

Abductor digiti
minimi muscle

Extensor digitorum
brevis muscle

PLATE **84b** SUPERFICIAL DISSECTION OF THE RIGHT FOOT,
LATERAL VIEW

Lateral malleolus

Extensor digitorum longus muscle

Tendons of extensor digitorum longus

Medial malleolus

Tendon of tibialis anterior

Site for palpation of dorsalis pedis artery

Dorsal venous arch

Tendon of extensor hallucis longus

PLATE **85a** SURFACE ANATOMY OF THE RIGHT FOOT, SUPERIOR VIEW

Fibularis brevis muscle

Superior extensor retinaculum

Lateral malleolus of fibula

Inferior extensor retinaculum

Tendons of extensor digitorum longus

Dorsal interosseus muscles

Tendons of extensor digitorum brevis

Medial malleolus of tibia

Tendon of tibialis anterior

Tendon of extensor hallucis longus

Abductor hallucis muscle

Tendon of extensor hallucis brevis

PLATE **85b** SUPERFICIAL DISSECTION OF THE RIGHT FOOT, SUPERIOR VIEW

Talus

Navicular

Cuboid

Cuneiform

Metatarsal bones (I-V)

Phalanges

Calcaneus

PLATE **86a** BONES OF THE RIGHT FOOT, LATERAL VIEW

Tibialis posterior muscle

Flexor hallucis longus

Calcaneal tendon

Talocalcaneal joint

Calcaneus

Navicular

Flexor digitorum, brevis muscle

Medial cuneiform bone

Plantar aponeurosis

Tibia

Talocrural joint

Subtalar joint

Talocalcaneal ligament

Talus

Talonavicular joint

Cuneonavicular joint

Tarsometatarsal joint

Metatarsal bone (II)

Adductor hallucis muscle

Metatarsophalangeal joint

Interphalangeal joint

PLATE **86c** MRI SCAN OF THE RIGHT ANKLE, SAGITTAL SECTION

Soleus muscle

Tibialis posterior

Calcaneal tendon

Talocalcaneal ligament

Quadratus plantae muscle

Calcaneus

Flexor digitorum brevis muscle

Flexor digitorum longus muscle

Tendon of tibialis anterior muscle

First cuneiform bone

Talus

Navicular bone

Base of first metatarsal bone

Flexor hallucis brevis muscle

TIBIA

PLATE **87a** ANKLE AND FOOT, POSTERIOR VIEW

Tendon of flexor digitorum longus muscle

Flexor hallucis longus muscle

Medial malleolus

Site for palpation of posterior tibial artery

Calcaneus

Tendon of fibularis longus muscle

Calcaneal tendon

Lateral malleolus

Tendon of fibularis brevis muscle

Base of fifth metatarsal bone

PLATE **87b** FRONTAL SECTION THROUGH THE RIGHT FOOT, POSTERIOR VIEW

Tibia

Talus

Medial malleolus

Deltoid ligament

Talocalcaneal ligament

Calcaneocuboid joint

Fibula

Talocrural (ankle) joint

Lateral malleolus

Calcaneus

Cuboid

PLATE **87c** MRI SCAN OF THE RIGHT ANKLE, FRONTAL SECTION

Extensor digitorum longus muscle

Tibia

Lateral malleolus of fibula

Talus

Calcaneus

Tendon of fibularis longus muscle

Abductor digiti minimi muscle

Medial malleolus of tibia

Tendon of tibialis posterior muscle

Deltoid ligament

Tendon of flexor digitorum longus muscle

Tendon of flexor hallucis longus muscle

Plantar artery

Abductor hallucis muscle

Quadratus plantae muscle

Flexor digitorum brevis muscle

Distal
phalanx

Distal phalanx

Proximal
phalanx

Middle phalanx

Proximal phalanx

Metatarsal
bones (I–V)

V   IV   III   II   I

Cuneiform
bones

Cuboid

Navicular

Talus

Calcaneus

Fibrous tendon
sheath

Tendons of flexor
digitorum brevis
muscle

Tendon of
flexor hallucis
longus muscle

Lumbrical
muscles

Flexor digiti
minimi muscle

Flexor hallucis
brevis muscle

Abductor
digiti minimi
muscle

Abductor hallucis
muscle

Flexor digitorum
brevis muscle

Plantar aponeurosis
(cut)

Calcaneus

PLATE **88** BONES OF THE RIGHT FOOT, INFERIOR
(PLANTAR) VIEW

PLATE **89** SUPERFICIAL DISSECTION OF THE RIGHT FOOT,
PLANTAR VIEW

Endochondral ossification replacing cartilages of embryonic skull

Intramembranous ossification producing the roofing bones of the skull

PLATE **90a** SKELETON OF FETUS AFTER **10** WEEKS OF DEVELOPMENT

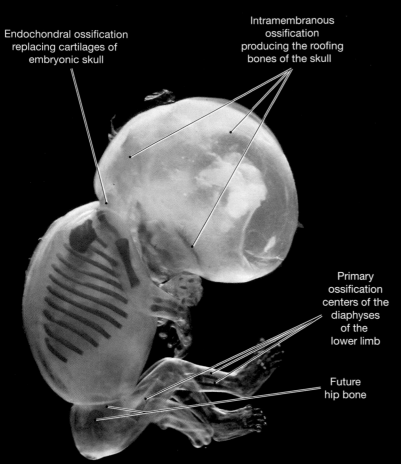

Primary ossification centers of the diaphyses of the lower limb

Future hip bone

Parietal bone

Temporal bone

Clavicle

Mandible

Frontal bone

Scapula

Humerus

Metacarpal bones

Phalanges

Ribs

Radius

Vertebrae

Ulna

Hip bone (ilium)

Cartilage of knee

Femur

Fibula

Tibia

Phalanx

Metatarsal bones

PLATE **90b** SKELETON OF FETUS AFTER **16** WEEKS OF DEVELOPMENT

Embryology Summaries

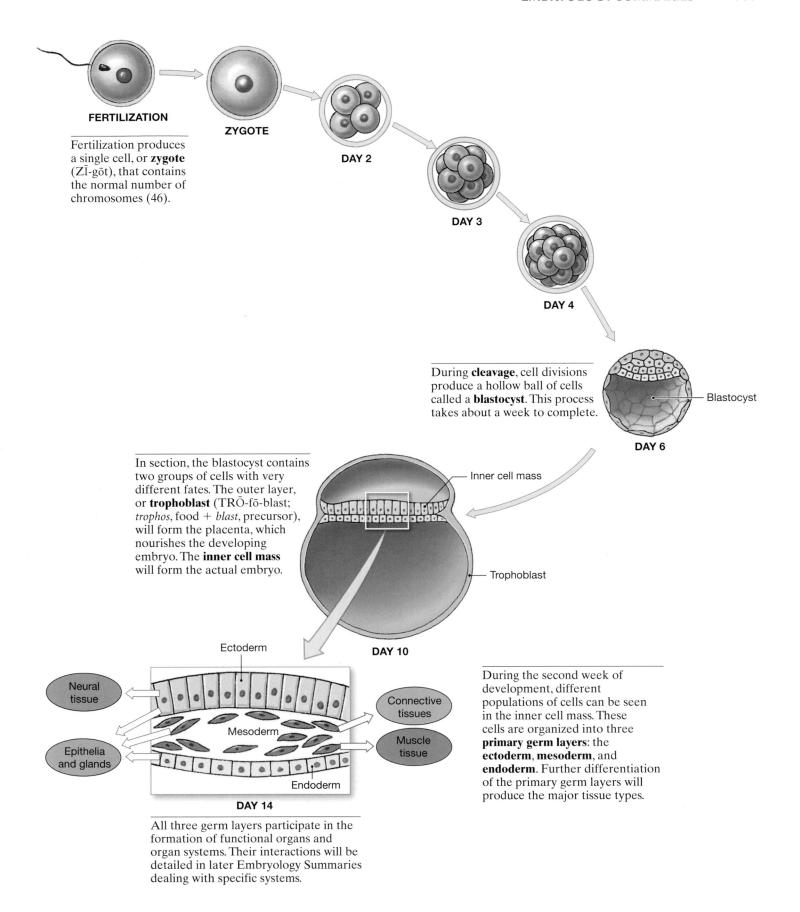

FERTILIZATION

Fertilization produces a single cell, or **zygote** (ZĪ-gōt), that contains the normal number of chromosomes (46).

ZYGOTE

DAY 2

DAY 3

DAY 4

During **cleavage**, cell divisions produce a hollow ball of cells called a **blastocyst**. This process takes about a week to complete.

Blastocyst

DAY 6

In section, the blastocyst contains two groups of cells with very different fates. The outer layer, or **trophoblast** (TRŌ-fō-blast; *trophos*, food + *blast*, precursor), will form the placenta, which nourishes the developing embryo. The **inner cell mass** will form the actual embryo.

Inner cell mass

Trophoblast

DAY 10

Ectoderm

Neural tissue

Connective tissues

Mesoderm

Muscle tissue

Epithelia and glands

Endoderm

DAY 14

During the second week of development, different populations of cells can be seen in the inner cell mass. These cells are organized into three **primary germ layers**: the **ectoderm**, **mesoderm**, and **endoderm**. Further differentiation of the primary germ layers will produce the major tissue types.

All three germ layers participate in the formation of functional organs and organ systems. Their interactions will be detailed in later Embryology Summaries dealing with specific systems.

EMBRYOLOGY SUMMARY **1:** THE FORMATION OF TISSUES

All epithelia begin as simple epithelia that may later become stratified.

These cells differentiate into functional epithelial cells and gland cells that may have endocrine or exocrine functions.

Epithelium

Connective tissue

Skin

Respiratory epithelium

Complex glands begin to form as epithelial cells grow into the underlying connective tissue.

Duct

In the formation of an **exocrine gland**, the cells connecting the secretory cells to the surface form the duct that carries the secretions of the gland cells to the epithelial surface.

Exocrine secretory cells

Connecting cells disappear

Blood vessel

In the formation of an **endocrine gland**, the connecting cells disappear, and the gland cells secrete into blood vessels or into the surrounding tissue fluids.

Endocrine secretory cells

EMBRYOLOGY SUMMARY 2: THE DEVELOPMENT OF EPITHELIA

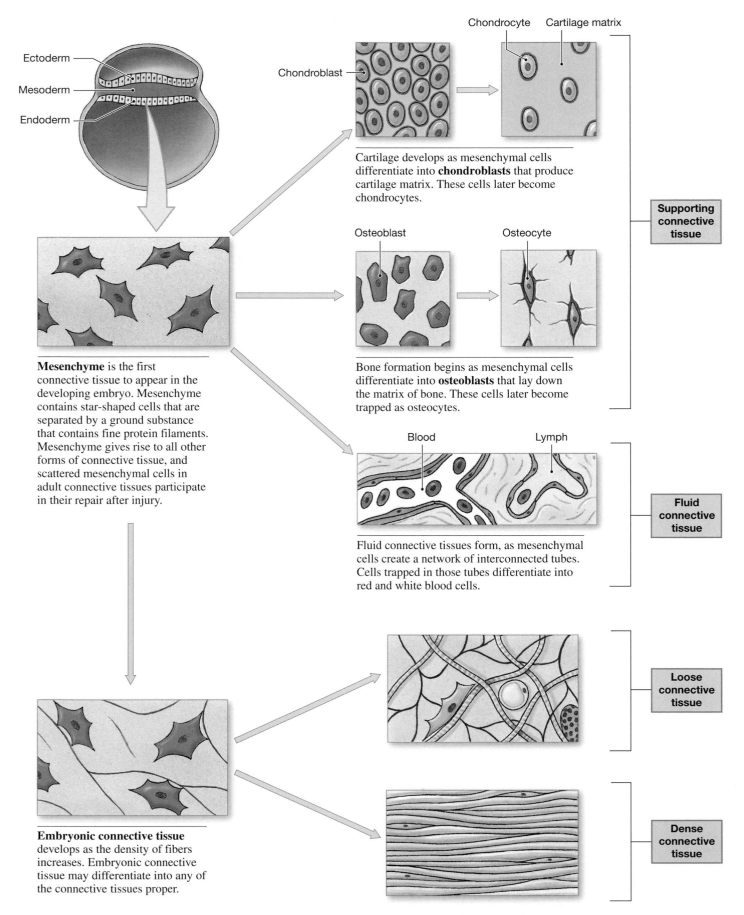

Ectoderm

Mesoderm

Endoderm

Chondroblast

Chondrocyte   Cartilage matrix

Cartilage develops as mesenchymal cells differentiate into **chondroblasts** that produce cartilage matrix. These cells later become chondrocytes.

Osteoblast

Osteocyte

Bone formation begins as mesenchymal cells differentiate into **osteoblasts** that lay down the matrix of bone. These cells later become trapped as osteocytes.

Blood

Lymph

Fluid connective tissues form, as mesenchymal cells create a network of interconnected tubes. Cells trapped in those tubes differentiate into red and white blood cells.

Mesenchyme is the first connective tissue to appear in the developing embryo. Mesenchyme contains star-shaped cells that are separated by a ground substance that contains fine protein filaments. Mesenchyme gives rise to all other forms of connective tissue, and scattered mesenchymal cells in adult connective tissues participate in their repair after injury.

Embryonic connective tissue develops as the density of fibers increases. Embryonic connective tissue may differentiate into any of the connective tissues proper.

Supporting connective tissue

Fluid connective tissue

Loose connective tissue

Dense connective tissue

EMBRYOLOGY SUMMARY **3**: THE ORIGINS OF CONNECTIVE TISSUES

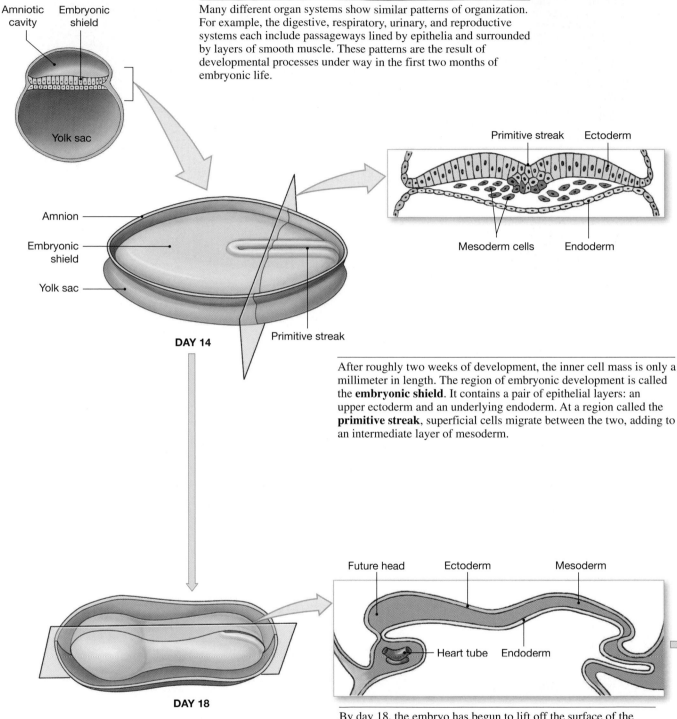

Amniotic cavity

Embryonic shield

Yolk sac

Many different organ systems show similar patterns of organization. For example, the digestive, respiratory, urinary, and reproductive systems each include passageways lined by epithelia and surrounded by layers of smooth muscle. These patterns are the result of developmental processes under way in the first two months of embryonic life.

Primitive streak Ectoderm

Mesoderm cells Endoderm

Amnion

Embryonic shield

Yolk sac

Primitive streak

DAY 14

After roughly two weeks of development, the inner cell mass is only a millimeter in length. The region of embryonic development is called the **embryonic shield**. It contains a pair of epithelial layers: an upper ectoderm and an underlying endoderm. At a region called the **primitive streak**, superficial cells migrate between the two, adding to an intermediate layer of mesoderm.

Future head Ectoderm Mesoderm

Heart tube Endoderm

DAY 18

By day 18, the embryo has begun to lift off the surface of the embryonic shield. The heart and many blood vessels have already formed, well ahead of the other organ systems. Unless otherwise noted, discussions of organ system development in subsequent Embryology Summaries will begin at this stage.

EMBRYOLOGY SUMMARY 4: THE DEVELOPMENT OF ORGAN SYSTEMS

DERIVATIVES OF PRIMARY GERM LAYERS

Ectoderm Forms: Epidermis and epidermal derivatives of the integumentary system, including hair follicles, nails, and glands communicating with the skin surface (sweat, milk, and sebum)
Lining of the mouth, salivary glands, nasal passageways, and anus
Nervous system, including brain and spinal cord
Portions of endocrine system (pituitary gland and parts of adrenal glands)
Portions of skull, pharyngeal arches, and teeth

Mesoderm Forms: Dermis of integumentary system
Lining of the body cavities (pleural, pericardial, peritoneal)
Muscular, skeletal, cardiovascular, and lymphatic systems
Kidneys and part of the urinary tract
Gonads and most of the reproductive tract
Connective tissues supporting all organ systems
Portions of endocrine system (parts of adrenal glands and endocrine tissues of the reproductive tract)

Endoderm Forms: Most of the digestive system: epithelium (except mouth and anus), exocrine glands (except salivary glands), the liver and pancreas
Most of the respiratory system: epithelium (except nasal passageways) and mucous glands
Portions of urinary and reproductive systems (ducts and the stem cells that produce gametes)
Portions of endocrine system (thymus, thyroid gland, parathyroid glands, and pancreas)

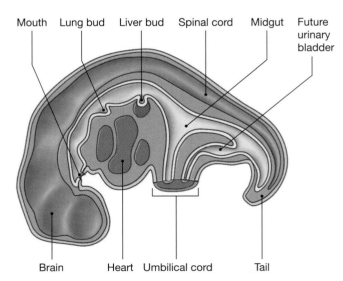

DAY 28

After one month, you can find the beginnings of all major organ systems. The role of each of the primary germ layers in the formation of organs is summarized in the accompanying table; details are given in later Embryology Summaries.

1 MONTH

At the start of the second month, the superficial ectoderm is a simple epithelium overlying loosely organized mesenchyme.

3 MONTHS

Over the following weeks, the epithelium becomes stratified through repeated divisions of the *basal* or *germinative cells*. The underlying mesenchyme differentiates into embryonic connective tissue containing blood vessels that bring nutrients to the region.

4 MONTHS

During the third and fourth months, small areas of epidermis undergo extensive divisions and form cords of cells that grow into the dermis. These are **epithelial columns**. Mesenchymal cells surround the columns as they extend deeper and deeper into the dermis. Hair follicles, sebaceous glands, and sweat glands develop from these columns.

SKIN

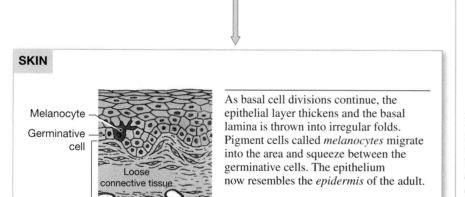

4 MONTHS

As basal cell divisions continue, the epithelial layer thickens and the basal lamina is thrown into irregular folds. Pigment cells called *melanocytes* migrate into the area and squeeze between the germinative cells. The epithelium now resembles the *epidermis* of the adult.

The embryonic connective tissue differentiates into the *dermis*. Fibroblasts and other connective tissue cells form from mesenchymal cells or migrate into the area. The density of fibers increases. Loose connective tissue extends into the ridges, but a deeper, less vascular region is dominated by a dense, irregular collagen fiber network. Below the dermis the embryonic connective tissue develops into the *subcutaneous layer*, a layer of loose connective tissue.

NAILS

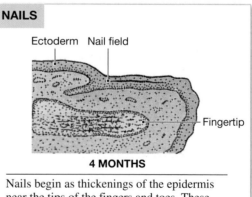

4 MONTHS

Nails begin as thickenings of the epidermis near the tips of the fingers and toes. These thickenings settle into the dermis, and the borderline with the general epidermis becomes distinct. Initially, nail production involves all of the germinative cells of the *nail field*.

BIRTH

By the time of birth, nail production is restricted to the *nail root*.

EMBRYOLOGY SUMMARY 5: THE DEVELOPMENT OF THE INTEGUMENTARY SYSTEM

HAIR FOLLICLES

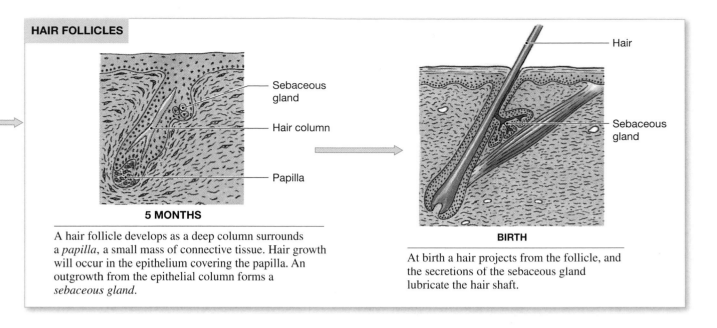

5 MONTHS

A hair follicle develops as a deep column surrounds a *papilla*, a small mass of connective tissue. Hair growth will occur in the epithelium covering the papilla. An outgrowth from the epithelial column forms a *sebaceous gland*.

BIRTH

At birth a hair projects from the follicle, and the secretions of the sebaceous gland lubricate the hair shaft.

EXOCRINE GLANDS

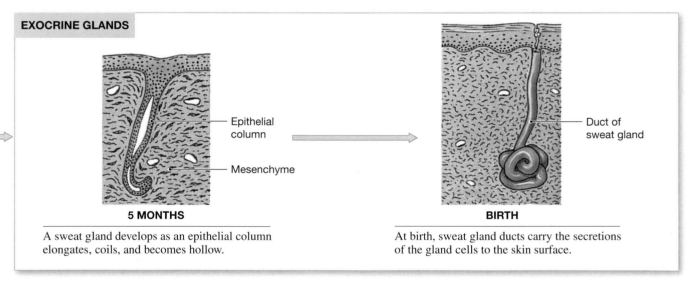

5 MONTHS

A sweat gland develops as an epithelial column elongates, coils, and becomes hollow.

BIRTH

At birth, sweat gland ducts carry the secretions of the gland cells to the skin surface.

MAMMARY GLANDS

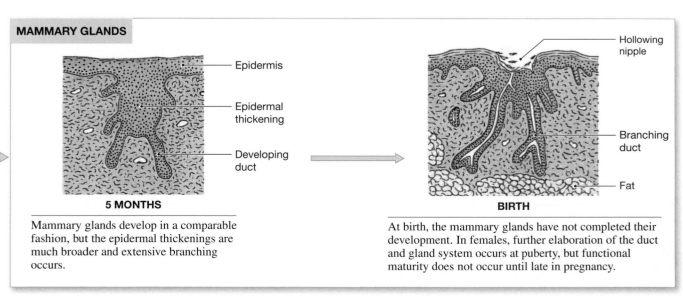

5 MONTHS

Mammary glands develop in a comparable fashion, but the epidermal thickenings are much broader and extensive branching occurs.

BIRTH

At birth, the mammary glands have not completed their development. In females, further elaboration of the duct and gland system occurs at puberty, but functional maturity does not occur until late in pregnancy.

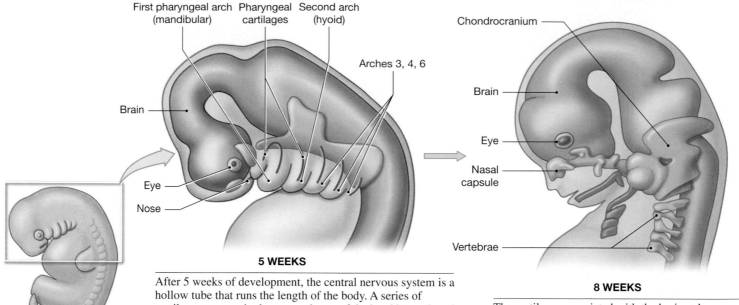

5-WEEK EMBRYO

5 WEEKS

After 5 weeks of development, the central nervous system is a hollow tube that runs the length of the body. A series of cartilages appears in the mesenchyme of the head beneath and alongside the expanding brain and around the developing nose, eyes, and ears. These cartilages are shown in light blue. Five additional pairs of cartilages develop in the walls of the pharynx. These cartilages, shown in dark blue, are located within the **pharyngeal**, or **branchial, arches**. (*Branchial* refers to gills—in fish the caudal arches develop into skeletal supports for the gills.) The first arch, or **mandibular arch**, is the largest.

8 WEEKS

The cartilages associated with the brain enlarge and fuse, forming a cartilaginous **chondrocranium** (kon-drō-KRĀ-nē-um; *chondros*, cartilage + *cranium*, skull) that cradles the brain and sense organs. At 8 weeks its walls and floor are incomplete, and there is no roof.

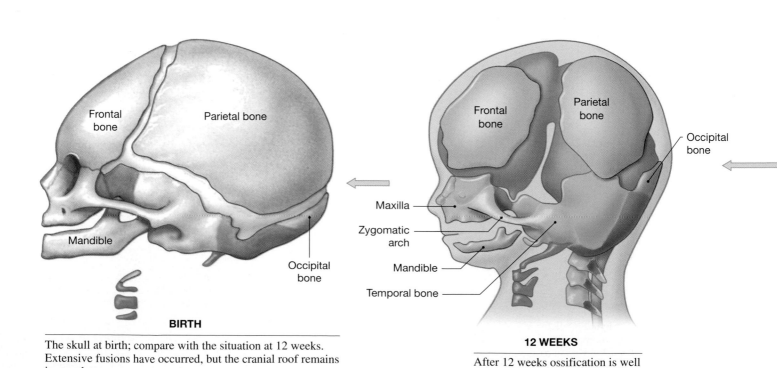

BIRTH

The skull at birth; compare with the situation at 12 weeks. Extensive fusions have occurred, but the cranial roof remains incomplete.

12 WEEKS

After 12 weeks ossification is well under way in the cranium and face. Compare with Plate 90b, page 114.

EMBRYOLOGY SUMMARY 6: THE DEVELOPMENT OF THE SKULL

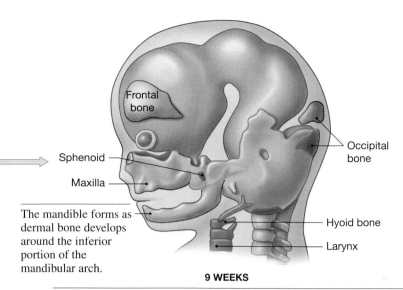

9 WEEKS

- Frontal bone
- Sphenoid
- Maxilla
- Occipital bone
- Hyoid bone
- Larynx

The mandible forms as dermal bone develops around the inferior portion of the mandibular arch.

During the ninth week, numerous centers of endochondral ossification appear within the chondrocranium. These centers are shown in red. Gradually, the frontal and parietal bones of the cranial roof appear as intramembranous ossification begins in the overlying dermis. As these centers (beige) enlarge and expand, extensive fusions occur.

The dorsal portion of the mandibular arch fuses with the chondrocranium. The fused cartilages do not ossify; instead, osteoblasts begin sheathing them in dermal bone. On each side this sheath fuses with a bone developing at the entrance to the nasal cavity, producing the two maxillae. Ossification centers in the roof of the mouth spread to form the palatine processes and later fuse with the maxillae.

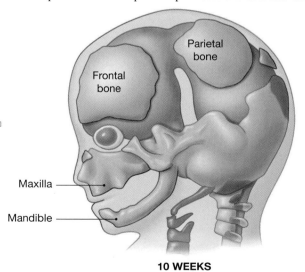

10 WEEKS

- Parietal bone
- Frontal bone
- Maxilla
- Mandible

The second arch, or **hyoid arch**, forms near the temporal bones. Fusion of the superior tips of the hyoid with the temporals forms the styloid processes. The ventral portion of the hyoid arch ossifies as the hyoid bone. The third arch fuses with the hyoid, and the fourth and sixth arches form laryngeal cartilages.

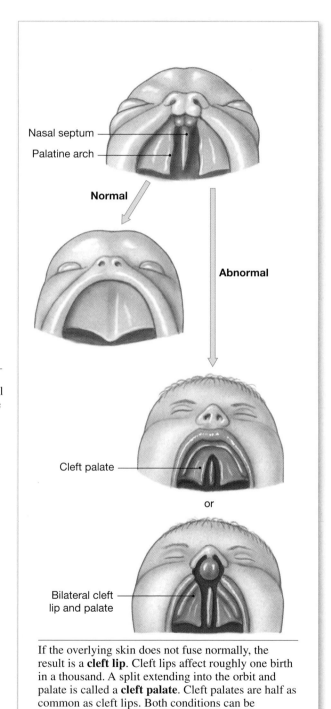

- Nasal septum
- Palatine arch

Normal

Abnormal

- Cleft palate

or

- Bilateral cleft lip and palate

If the overlying skin does not fuse normally, the result is a **cleft lip**. Cleft lips affect roughly one birth in a thousand. A split extending into the orbit and palate is called a **cleft palate**. Cleft palates are half as common as cleft lips. Both conditions can be corrected surgically.

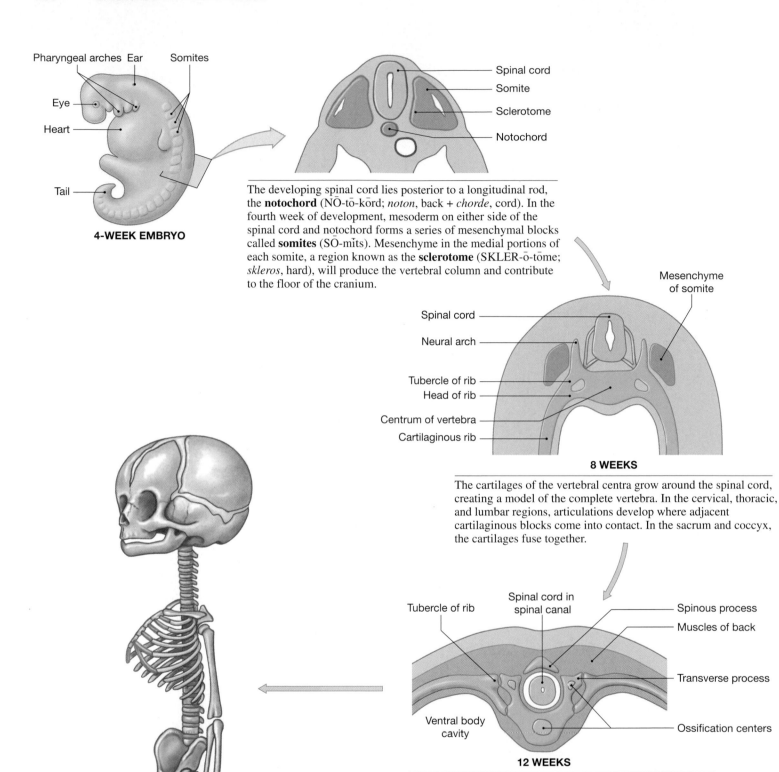

Pharyngeal arches Ear Somites

Eye

Heart

Tail

4-WEEK EMBRYO

Spinal cord
Somite
Sclerotome
Notochord

The developing spinal cord lies posterior to a longitudinal rod, the **notochord** (NŌ-tō-kōrd; *noton*, back + *chorde*, cord). In the fourth week of development, mesoderm on either side of the spinal cord and notochord forms a series of mesenchymal blocks called **somites** (SŌ-mĭts). Mesenchyme in the medial portions of each somite, a region known as the **sclerotome** (SKLER-ō-tōme; *skleros*, hard), will produce the vertebral column and contribute to the floor of the cranium.

Mesenchyme of somite

Spinal cord
Neural arch

Tubercle of rib
Head of rib
Centrum of vertebra
Cartilaginous rib

8 WEEKS

The cartilages of the vertebral centra grow around the spinal cord, creating a model of the complete vertebra. In the cervical, thoracic, and lumbar regions, articulations develop where adjacent cartilaginous blocks come into contact. In the sacrum and coccyx, the cartilages fuse together.

Tubercle of rib

Spinal cord in spinal canal

Spinous process
Muscles of back

Transverse process

Ventral body cavity

Ossification centers

12 WEEKS

About the time the ribs separate from the vertebrae, ossification begins. Only the shortest ribs undergo complete ossification. In the rest, the distal portions remain cartilaginous, forming the costal cartilages. Several ossification centers appear in the sternum, but fusion gradually reduces the number.

BIRTH

At birth, the vertebrae and ribs are ossified, but many cartilaginous areas remain. For example, the anterior portions of the ribs remain cartilaginous. Additional growth will occur for many years; in vertebrae, the bases of the neural arches enlarge until ages 3–6, and the spinal processes and vertebral bodies grow until ages 18–25.

EMBRYOLOGY SUMMARY **7:** THE DEVELOPMENT OF THE VERTEBRAL COLUMN

4 WEEKS

Cells of the sclerotomal segments migrate away from the somites and cluster around the notochord.

6 WEEKS

The migrating cells differentiate into chondroblasts and produce a series of cartilaginous blocks that surround the notochord. These cartilages, which will develop into the vertebral centra, are separated by patches of mesenchyme.

8 WEEKS

ADULT

Expansion of the vertebral centra eventually eliminates the notochord, but it remains intact between adjacent vertebrae, forming the *nucleus pulposus* of the intervertebral discs. Later, surrounding mesenchymal cells differentiate into chondroblasts and produce the fibrous cartilage of the *anulus fibrosus*.

8 WEEKS

9 WEEKS

Rib cartilages expand away from the developing transverse processes of the vertebrae. At first they are continuous, but by week 8 the ribs have separated from the vertebrae. Ribs form at every vertebra, but in the cervical, lumbar, sacral, and coccygeal regions they remain small and later fuse with the growing vertebrae. The ribs of the thoracic vertebrae continue to enlarge, following the curvature of the body wall. When they reach the ventral midline, they fuse with the cartilages of the sternum.

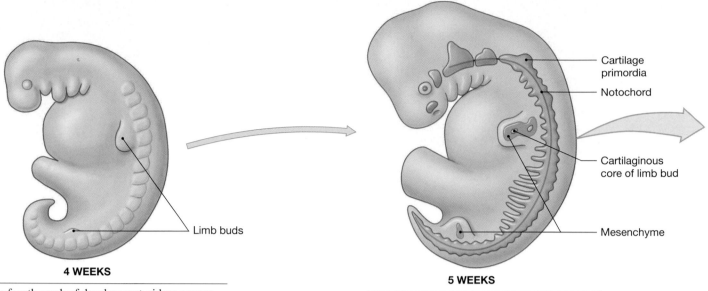

4 WEEKS

In the fourth week of development, ridges appear along the flanks of the embryo, extending from just behind the throat to just before the anus. These ridges form as mesodermal cells congregate beneath the ectoderm of the flank. Mesoderm gradually accumulates at the end of each ridge, forming two pairs of limb buds.

5 WEEKS

After 5 weeks of development, the pectoral limb buds have a cartilaginous core and scapular cartilages are developing in the mesenchyme of the trunk.

BIRTH

The skeleton of a newborn infant. Note the extensive areas of cartilage (blue) in the humeral head, in the wrist, between the bones of the palm and fingers, and in the hips. Notice the appearance of the axial skeleton, with reference to the two previous Embryology Summaries.

10 WEEKS

Ossification in the embryonic skeleton after approximately 10 weeks of development. The shafts of the limb bones are undergoing rapid ossification, but the distal bones of the carpus and tarsus remain cartilaginous.

EMBRYOLOGY SUMMARY 8: THE DEVELOPMENT OF THE APPENDICULAR SKELETON

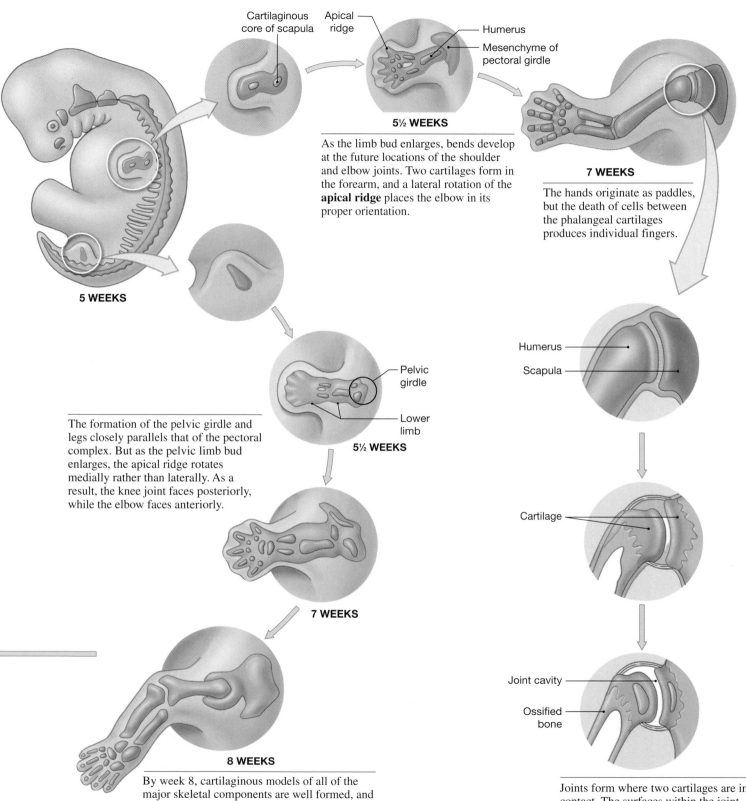

Cartilaginous core of scapula

Apical ridge

Humerus

Mesenchyme of pectoral girdle

5½ WEEKS

As the limb bud enlarges, bends develop at the future locations of the shoulder and elbow joints. Two cartilages form in the forearm, and a lateral rotation of the **apical ridge** places the elbow in its proper orientation.

7 WEEKS

The hands originate as paddles, but the death of cells between the phalangeal cartilages produces individual fingers.

5 WEEKS

Pelvic girdle

Lower limb

5½ WEEKS

The formation of the pelvic girdle and legs closely parallels that of the pectoral complex. But as the pelvic limb bud enlarges, the apical ridge rotates medially rather than laterally. As a result, the knee joint faces posteriorly, while the elbow faces anteriorly.

Humerus

Scapula

Cartilage

7 WEEKS

Joint cavity

Ossified bone

8 WEEKS

By week 8, cartilaginous models of all of the major skeletal components are well formed, and endochondral ossification begins in the future limb bones. Ossification of the hip bones begins at three separate centers that gradually enlarge.

Joints form where two cartilages are in contact. The surfaces within the joint cavity remain cartilaginous, while the rest of the bones undergo ossification.

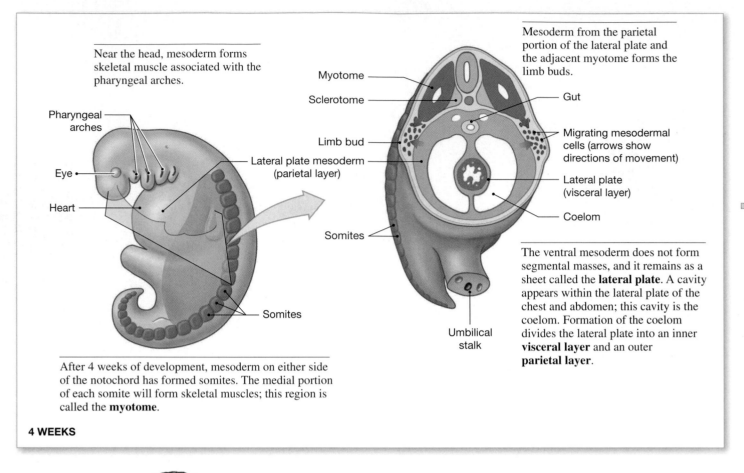

Near the head, mesoderm forms skeletal muscle associated with the pharyngeal arches.

Mesoderm from the parietal portion of the lateral plate and the adjacent myotome forms the limb buds.

After 4 weeks of development, mesoderm on either side of the notochord has formed somites. The medial portion of each somite will form skeletal muscles; this region is called the **myotome**.

The ventral mesoderm does not form segmental masses, and it remains as a sheet called the **lateral plate**. A cavity appears within the lateral plate of the chest and abdomen; this cavity is the coelom. Formation of the coelom divides the lateral plate into an inner **visceral layer** and an outer **parietal layer**.

4 WEEKS

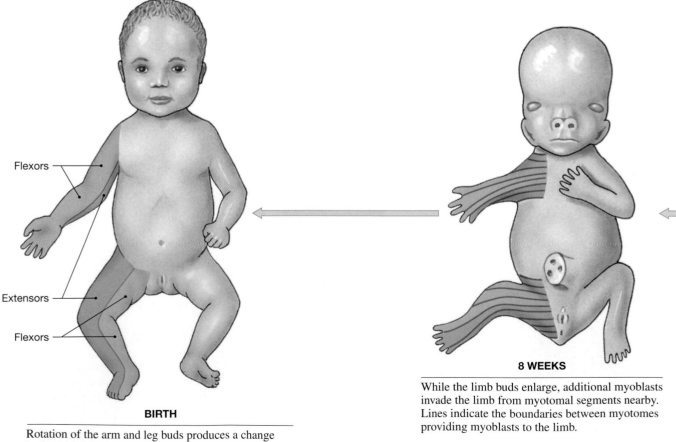

BIRTH

Rotation of the arm and leg buds produces a change in the position of these masses relative to the body axis.

8 WEEKS

While the limb buds enlarge, additional myoblasts invade the limb from myotomal segments nearby. Lines indicate the boundaries between myotomes providing myoblasts to the limb.

EMBRYOLOGY SUMMARY 9: THE DEVELOPMENT OF THE MUSCULAR SYSTEM

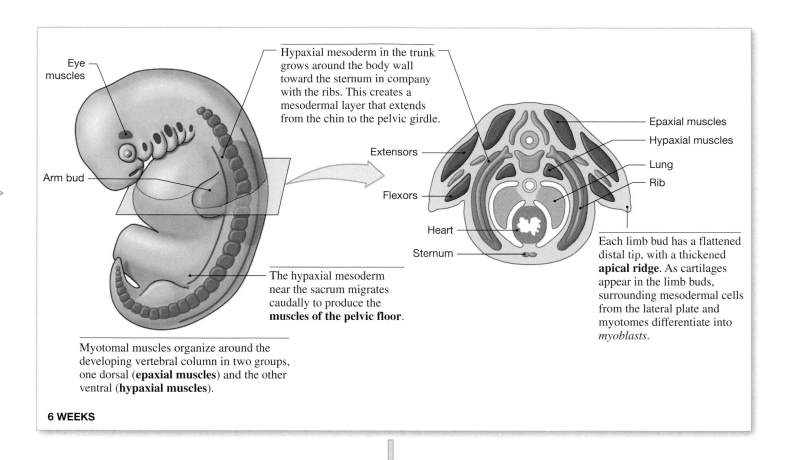

Eye muscles

Hypaxial mesoderm in the trunk grows around the body wall toward the sternum in company with the ribs. This creates a mesodermal layer that extends from the chin to the pelvic girdle.

Arm bud

Epaxial muscles

Hypaxial muscles

Extensors

Lung

Rib

Flexors

Heart

The hypaxial mesoderm near the sacrum migrates caudally to produce the **muscles of the pelvic floor**.

Sternum

Each limb bud has a flattened distal tip, with a thickened **apical ridge**. As cartilages appear in the limb buds, surrounding mesodermal cells from the lateral plate and myotomes differentiate into *myoblasts*.

Myotomal muscles organize around the developing vertebral column in two groups, one dorsal (**epaxial muscles**) and the other ventral (**hypaxial muscles**).

6 WEEKS

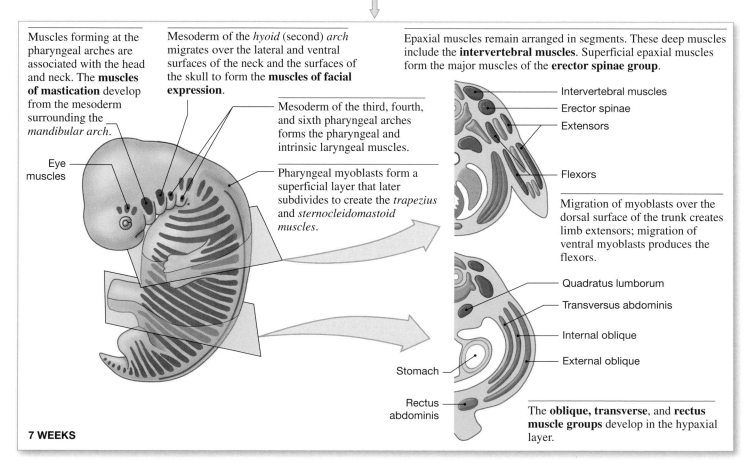

Muscles forming at the pharyngeal arches are associated with the head and neck. The **muscles of mastication** develop from the mesoderm surrounding the *mandibular arch*.

Mesoderm of the *hyoid* (second) *arch* migrates over the lateral and ventral surfaces of the neck and the surfaces of the skull to form the **muscles of facial expression**.

Epaxial muscles remain arranged in segments. These deep muscles include the **intervertebral muscles**. Superficial epaxial muscles form the major muscles of the **erector spinae group**.

Mesoderm of the third, fourth, and sixth pharyngeal arches forms the pharyngeal and intrinsic laryngeal muscles.

Intervertebral muscles

Erector spinae

Extensors

Eye muscles

Pharyngeal myoblasts form a superficial layer that later subdivides to create the *trapezius* and *sternocleidomastoid muscles*.

Flexors

Migration of myoblasts over the dorsal surface of the trunk creates limb extensors; migration of ventral myoblasts produces the flexors.

Quadratus lumborum

Transversus abdominis

Internal oblique

External oblique

Stomach

Rectus abdominis

The **oblique, transverse**, and **rectus muscle groups** develop in the hypaxial layer.

7 WEEKS

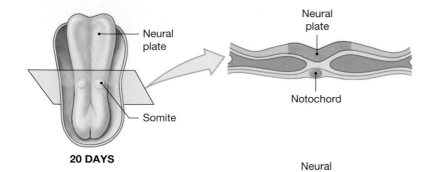

20 DAYS

After two weeks of development, *somites* are appearing on either side of the *notochord*. The ectoderm near the midline thickens, forming an elevated neural plate. The **neural plate** is largest near the future head of the developing embryo.

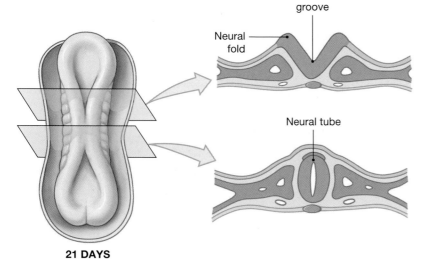

21 DAYS

A crease develops along the axis of the neural plate, creating the **neural groove**. The edges, or **neural folds**, gradually move together. They first contact one another midway along the axis of the neural plate, near the end of the third week.

Where the neural folds meet, they fuse to form a cylindrical **neural tube** that loses its connection with the superficial ectoderm. The process of neural tube formation is called **neurulation**; it is completed in less than a week. The formation of the axial skeleton and that of the musculature around the developing neural tube were described on pages 126–127 and 130–131.

Cells at the tips of the neural folds do not participate in neural tube formation. These cells of the **neural crest** at first remain between the dorsal surface of the neural tube and the ectoderm, but they later migrate to other locations. The neural tube becomes the CNS. Axons from neurons within the neural tube and the axons of neural crest cells form the PNS.

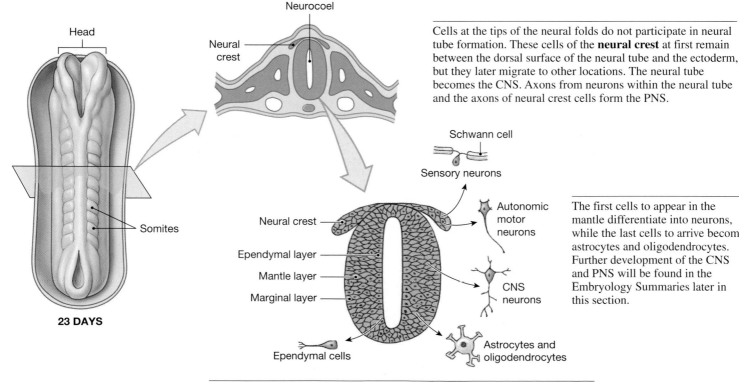

23 DAYS

The first cells to appear in the mantle differentiate into neurons, while the last cells to arrive become astrocytes and oligodendrocytes. Further development of the CNS and PNS will be found in the Embryology Summaries later in this section.

The neural tube increases in thickness as its epithelial lining undergoes repeated mitoses. By the middle of the fifth developmental week, there are three distinct layers. The **ependymal layer** lines the enclosed cavity, or **neurocoel**. The ependymal cells continue their mitotic activities, and daughter cells create the surrounding **mantle layer**. Axons from developing neurons form a superficial **marginal layer**.

EMBRYOLOGY SUMMARY **10:** AN INTRODUCTION TO THE DEVELOPMENT OF THE NERVOUS SYSTEM

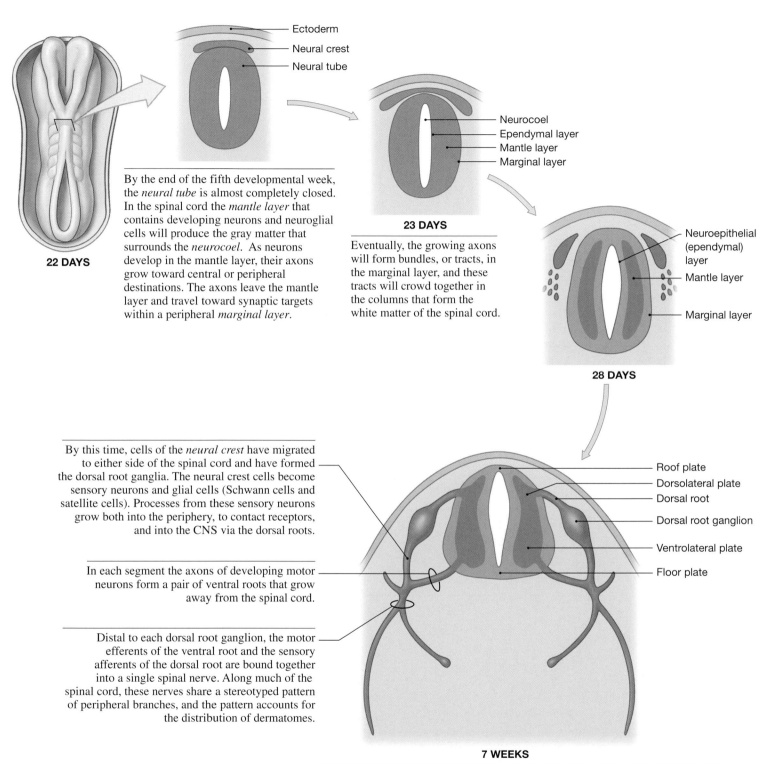

22 DAYS

Ectoderm
Neural crest
Neural tube

23 DAYS

Neurocoel
Ependymal layer
Mantle layer
Marginal layer

By the end of the fifth developmental week, the *neural tube* is almost completely closed. In the spinal cord the *mantle layer* that contains developing neurons and neuroglial cells will produce the gray matter that surrounds the *neurocoel*. As neurons develop in the mantle layer, their axons grow toward central or peripheral destinations. The axons leave the mantle layer and travel toward synaptic targets within a peripheral *marginal layer*.

Eventually, the growing axons will form bundles, or tracts, in the marginal layer, and these tracts will crowd together in the columns that form the white matter of the spinal cord.

28 DAYS

Neuroepithelial (ependymal) layer
Mantle layer
Marginal layer

By this time, cells of the *neural crest* have migrated to either side of the spinal cord and have formed the dorsal root ganglia. The neural crest cells become sensory neurons and glial cells (Schwann cells and satellite cells). Processes from these sensory neurons grow both into the periphery, to contact receptors, and into the CNS via the dorsal roots.

In each segment the axons of developing motor neurons form a pair of ventral roots that grow away from the spinal cord.

Distal to each dorsal root ganglion, the motor efferents of the ventral root and the sensory afferents of the dorsal root are bound together into a single spinal nerve. Along much of the spinal cord, these nerves share a stereotyped pattern of peripheral branches, and the pattern accounts for the distribution of dermatomes.

Roof plate
Dorsolateral plate
Dorsal root
Dorsal root ganglion
Ventrolateral plate
Floor plate

7 WEEKS

As the mantle enlarges, the neurocoel becomes laterally compressed and relatively narrow. The relatively thin **roof plate** and **floor plate** will not thicken substantially, but the **dorsolateral** and **ventrolateral plates** enlarge rapidly. Neurons developing within the dorsolateral plate will receive and relay sensory information, while those in the ventrolateral region will develop into motor neurons.

EMBRYOLOGY SUMMARY 11: THE DEVELOPMENT OF THE SPINAL CORD AND SPINAL NERVES—PART I

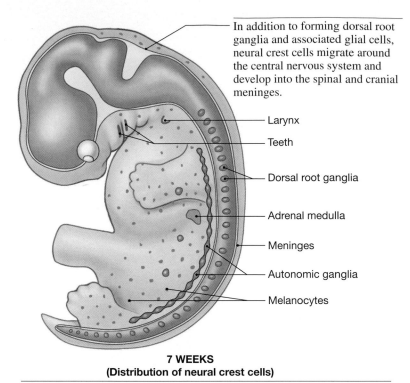

In addition to forming dorsal root ganglia and associated glial cells, neural crest cells migrate around the central nervous system and develop into the spinal and cranial meninges.

- Larynx
- Teeth
- Dorsal root ganglia
- Adrenal medulla
- Meninges
- Autonomic ganglia
- Melanocytes

7 WEEKS
(Distribution of neural crest cells)

Neural crest cells aggregate to form autonomic ganglia near the vertebral column and in peripheral organs. Migrating neural crest cells contribute to the formation of teeth and form the laryngeal cartilages, melanocytes of the skin, the skull, connective tissues around the eye, the intrinsic muscles of the eye, Schwann cells, satellite cells, and the adrenal medullae.

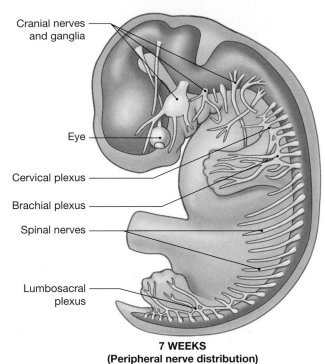

- Cranial nerves and ganglia
- Eye
- Cervical plexus
- Brachial plexus
- Spinal nerves
- Lumbosacral plexus

7 WEEKS
(Peripheral nerve distribution)

Several spinal nerves innervate each developing limb. When embryonic muscle cells migrate away from the myotome, the nerves grow right along with them. If a large muscle in the adult is derived from several myotomal blocks, connective tissue partitions will often mark the original boundaries, and the innervation will always involve more than one spinal nerve.

DEVELOPMENTAL ABNORMALITIES

Spina bifida

Neural tube defect

Spina bifida (BI-fi-da) results when the developing vertebral laminae fail to unite due to abnormal neural tube formation at that site. The neural arch is incomplete, and the meninges bulge outward beneath the skin of the back. The extent of the abnormality determines the severity of the defects. In mild cases, the condition may pass unnoticed; extreme cases involve much of the length of the vertebral column.

A **neural tube defect (NTD)** is a condition that is secondary to a developmental error in the formation of the spinal cord. Instead of forming a hollow tube, a portion of the spinal cord develops as a broad plate. This is often associated with spina bifida. Neural tube defects affect roughly one individual in 1000; prenatal testing can detect the existence of these defects with an 80–85 percent success rate.

EMBRYOLOGY SUMMARY 11: THE DEVELOPMENT OF THE SPINAL CORD AND SPINAL NERVES—*PART II*

Before proceeding, briefly review the summaries of skull formation, vertebral column development, and development of the spinal cord in the previous Embryology Summaries.

The initial cephalic expansion occurs as the neurocoel enlarges, forming three distinct **brain vesicles**: (1) the **prosencephalon** (prōs-en-SEF-a-lon) or "forebrain," (2) the **mesencephalon** or "midbrain," and (3) the **rhombencephalon** (rom-ben-SEF-a-lon) or "hindbrain." The prosencephalon and rhombencephalon will be subdivided further as development proceeds.

Even before **neural tube** formation has been completed, the cephalic portion begins to enlarge. Major differences in brain versus spinal cord development include (1) early breakdown of mantle (gray matter) and marginal (white matter) organization; (2) appearance of areas of neural cortex; (3) differential growth between and within specific regions; (4) appearance of characteristic bends and folds; and (5) loss of obvious segmental organization.

23 DAYS

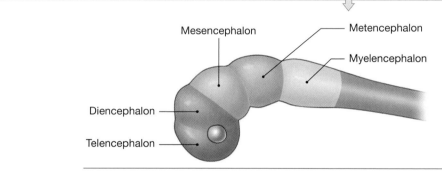

The rhombencephalon first subdivides into the **metencephalon** (met-en-SEF-a-lon; *meta*, after) and the **myelencephalon** (mi-el-ēn-SEF-a-lon; *myelon*, spinal cord).

The prosencephalon forms the **telecephalon** (tel-en-SEF-a-lon; *telos*, end + *enkephalos*, brain) and the **diencephalon**. The telencephalon begins as a pair of swellings near the rostral, dorsolateral border of the prosencephalon.

4 WEEKS

Cranial nerves develop as sensory ganglia and link peripheral receptors with the brain, and motor fibers grow out of developing cranial nuclei. Special sensory neurons of cranial nerves N I, II, and VIII develop in association with the developing receptors. The somatic motor nerves (N III, IV, and VI) grow to the eye muscles; the mixed nerves (N V, VII, IX, and X) innervate the **pharyngeal arches**.

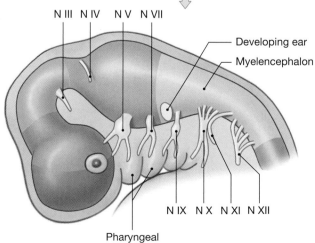

Development of the **mesencephalon** produces a small mass of neural tissue with a constricted neurocoel, the *aqueduct of the midbrain*.

As differential growth proceeds and the position and orientation of the embryo change, a series of bends, or **flexures** (FLEK-sherz), appears along the axis of the developing brain.

5 WEEKS

EMBRYOLOGY SUMMARY 12: THE DEVELOPMENT OF THE BRAIN AND CRANIAL NERVES—PART I

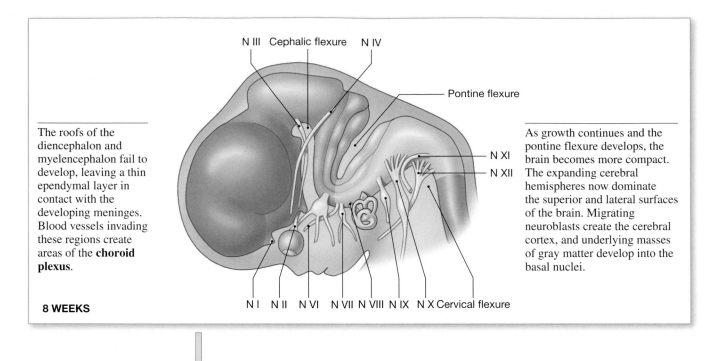

The roofs of the diencephalon and myelencephalon fail to develop, leaving a thin ependymal layer in contact with the developing meninges. Blood vessels invading these regions create areas of the **choroid plexus**.

8 WEEKS

As growth continues and the pontine flexure develops, the brain becomes more compact. The expanding cerebral hemispheres now dominate the superior and lateral surfaces of the brain. Migrating neuroblasts create the cerebral cortex, and underlying masses of gray matter develop into the basal nuclei.

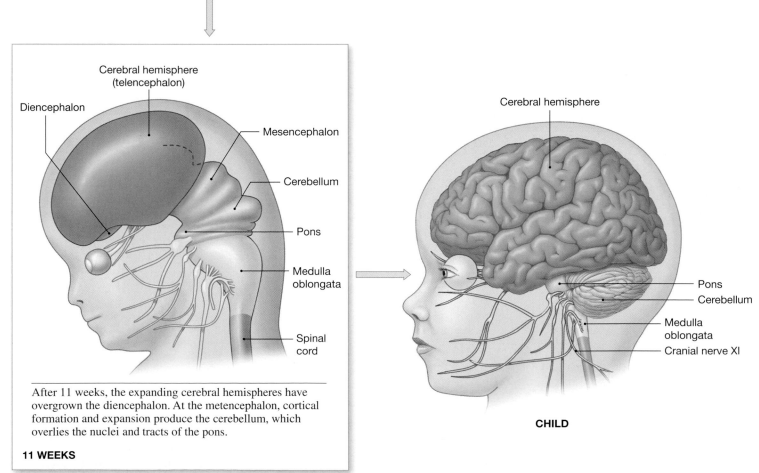

After 11 weeks, the expanding cerebral hemispheres have overgrown the diencephalon. At the metencephalon, cortical formation and expansion produce the cerebellum, which overlies the nuclei and tracts of the pons.

11 WEEKS

CHILD

EMBRYOLOGY SUMMARY 12: THE DEVELOPMENT OF THE BRAIN AND CRANIAL NERVES—PART II

All special sense organs develop from the interaction between the epithelia and the developing nervous system of the embryo.

VISION

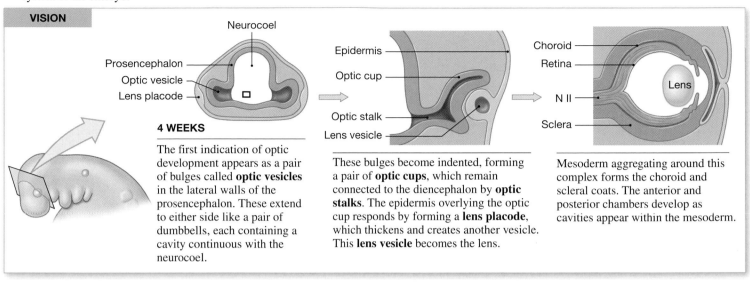

4 WEEKS

The first indication of optic development appears as a pair of bulges called **optic vesicles** in the lateral walls of the prosencephalon. These extend to either side like a pair of dumbbells, each containing a cavity continuous with the neurocoel.

These bulges become indented, forming a pair of **optic cups**, which remain connected to the diencephalon by **optic stalks**. The epidermis overlying the optic cup responds by forming a **lens placode**, which thickens and creates another vesicle. This **lens vesicle** becomes the lens.

Mesoderm aggregating around this complex forms the choroid and scleral coats. The anterior and posterior chambers develop as cavities appear within the mesoderm.

OLFACTION

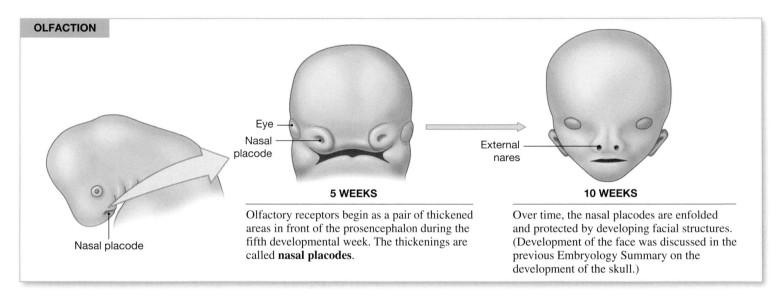

5 WEEKS

Olfactory receptors begin as a pair of thickened areas in front of the prosencephalon during the fifth developmental week. The thickenings are called **nasal placodes**.

10 WEEKS

Over time, the nasal placodes are enfolded and protected by developing facial structures. (Development of the face was discussed in the previous Embryology Summary on the development of the skull.)

GUSTATION

Gustatory receptors are the least specialized of any of the special sense organs. Taste buds develop as sensory fibers grow into the developing mouth and pharynx.

When the nerve endings contact epithelial cells, the epithelial cells differentiate into gustatory cells. If the sensory nerves are cut, the taste buds degenerate; if the sensory nerve is moved, it will stimulate the development of new taste buds at its new location.

EMBRYOLOGY SUMMARY 13: THE DEVELOPMENT OF SPECIAL SENSE ORGANS—PART I

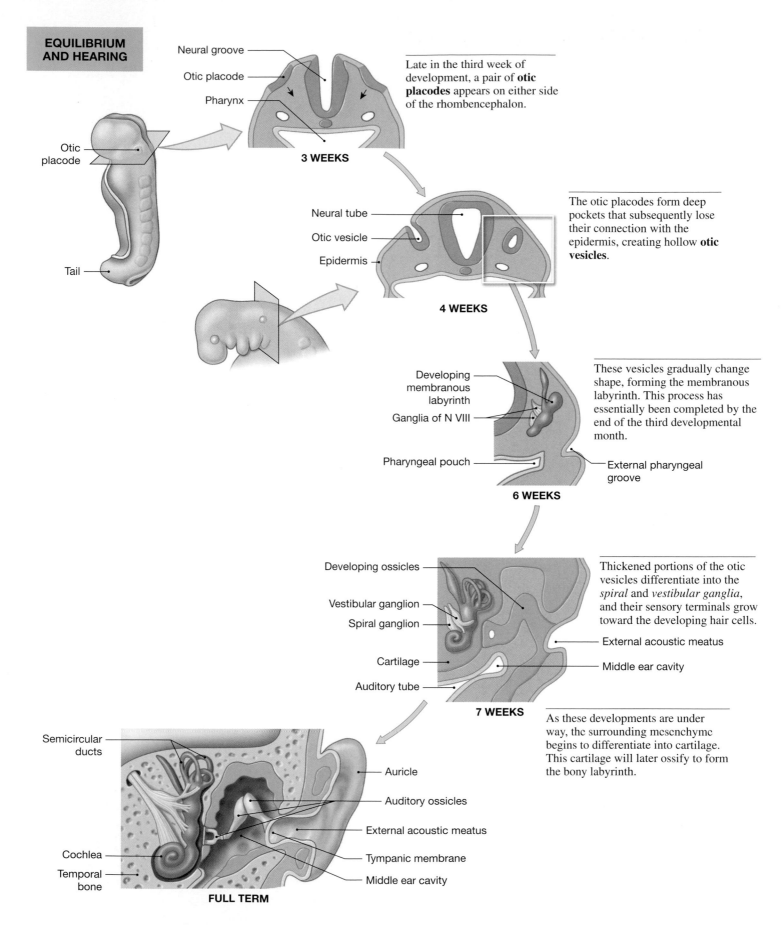

EQUILIBRIUM AND HEARING

Neural groove

Otic placode

Pharynx

Otic placode

Tail

3 WEEKS

Late in the third week of development, a pair of **otic placodes** appears on either side of the rhombencephalon.

Neural tube

Otic vesicle

Epidermis

4 WEEKS

The otic placodes form deep pockets that subsequently lose their connection with the epidermis, creating hollow **otic vesicles**.

Developing membranous labyrinth

Ganglia of N VIII

Pharyngeal pouch

External pharyngeal groove

6 WEEKS

These vesicles gradually change shape, forming the membranous labyrinth. This process has essentially been completed by the end of the third developmental month.

Developing ossicles

Vestibular ganglion

Spiral ganglion

Cartilage

Auditory tube

External acoustic meatus

Middle ear cavity

7 WEEKS

Thickened portions of the otic vesicles differentiate into the *spiral* and *vestibular ganglia*, and their sensory terminals grow toward the developing hair cells.

As these developments are under way, the surrounding mesenchyme begins to differentiate into cartilage. This cartilage will later ossify to form the bony labyrinth.

Semicircular ducts

Auricle

Auditory ossicles

External acoustic meatus

Cochlea

Tympanic membrane

Temporal bone

Middle ear cavity

FULL TERM

EMBRYOLOGY SUMMARY 13: THE DEVELOPMENT OF SPECIAL SENSE ORGANS—PART II

All secretory glands, whether exocrine or endocrine, are derived from epithelia. Endocrine organs develop from epithelia (1) covering the outside of the embryo, (2) lining the digestive tract, and (3) lining the coelomic cavity.

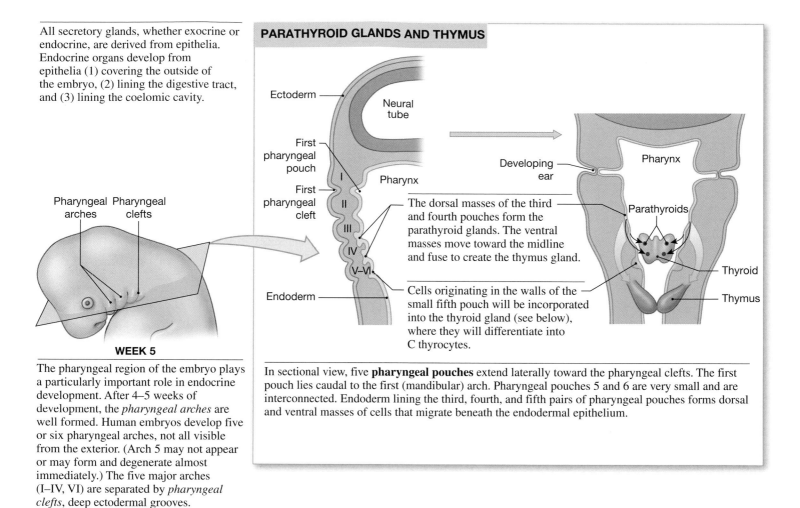

PARATHYROID GLANDS AND THYMUS

The dorsal masses of the third and fourth pouches form the parathyroid glands. The ventral masses move toward the midline and fuse to create the thymus gland.

Cells originating in the walls of the small fifth pouch will be incorporated into the thyroid gland (see below), where they will differentiate into C thyrocytes.

WEEK 5

The pharyngeal region of the embryo plays a particularly important role in endocrine development. After 4–5 weeks of development, the *pharyngeal arches* are well formed. Human embryos develop five or six pharyngeal arches, not all visible from the exterior. (Arch 5 may not appear or may form and degenerate almost immediately.) The five major arches (I–IV, VI) are separated by *pharyngeal clefts*, deep ectodermal grooves.

In sectional view, five **pharyngeal pouches** extend laterally toward the pharyngeal clefts. The first pouch lies caudal to the first (mandibular) arch. Pharyngeal pouches 5 and 6 are very small and are interconnected. Endoderm lining the third, fourth, and fifth pairs of pharyngeal pouches forms dorsal and ventral masses of cells that migrate beneath the endodermal epithelium.

THYROID GLAND

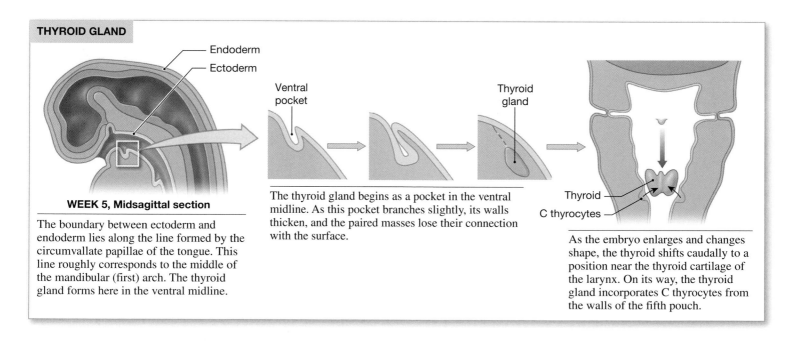

WEEK 5, Midsagittal section

The boundary between ectoderm and endoderm lies along the line formed by the circumvallate papillae of the tongue. This line roughly corresponds to the middle of the mandibular (first) arch. The thyroid gland forms here in the ventral midline.

The thyroid gland begins as a pocket in the ventral midline. As this pocket branches slightly, its walls thicken, and the paired masses lose their connection with the surface.

As the embryo enlarges and changes shape, the thyroid shifts caudally to a position near the thyroid cartilage of the larynx. On its way, the thyroid gland incorporates C thyrocytes from the walls of the fifth pouch.

EMBRYOLOGY SUMMARY **14**: THE DEVELOPMENT OF THE ENDOCRINE SYSTEM—*PART I*

PITUITARY GLAND

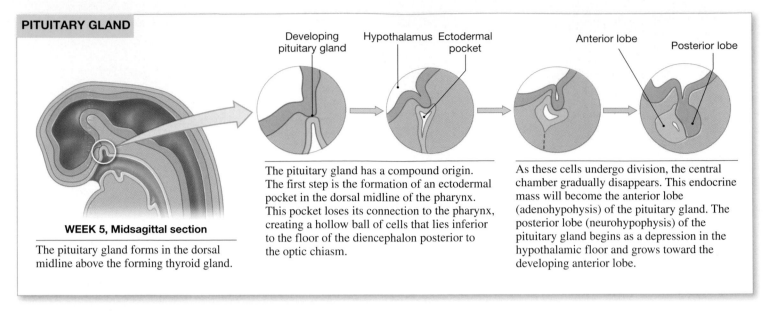

WEEK 5, Midsagittal section

The pituitary gland forms in the dorsal midline above the forming thyroid gland.

The pituitary gland has a compound origin. The first step is the formation of an ectodermal pocket in the dorsal midline of the pharynx. This pocket loses its connection to the pharynx, creating a hollow ball of cells that lies inferior to the floor of the diencephalon posterior to the optic chiasm.

As these cells undergo division, the central chamber gradually disappears. This endocrine mass will become the anterior lobe (adenohypophysis) of the pituitary gland. The posterior lobe (neurohypophysis) of the pituitary gland begins as a depression in the hypothalamic floor and grows toward the developing anterior lobe.

ADRENAL GLANDS

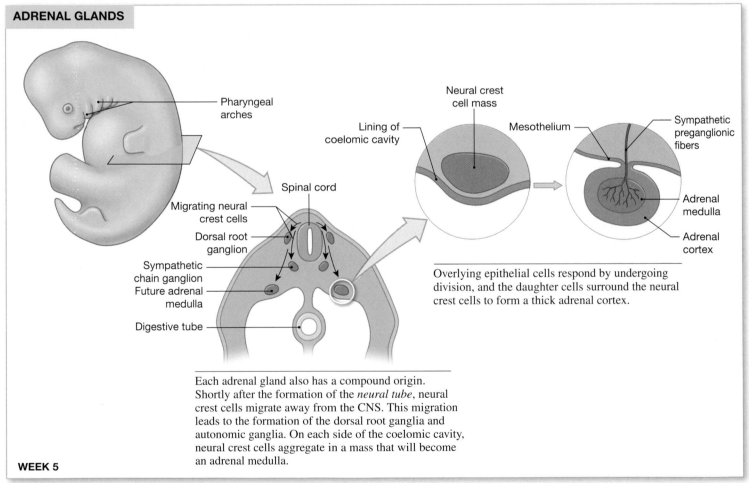

Overlying epithelial cells respond by undergoing division, and the daughter cells surround the neural crest cells to form a thick adrenal cortex.

Each adrenal gland also has a compound origin. Shortly after the formation of the *neural tube*, neural crest cells migrate away from the CNS. This migration leads to the formation of the dorsal root ganglia and autonomic ganglia. On each side of the coelomic cavity, neural crest cells aggregate in a mass that will become an adrenal medulla.

WEEK 5

For additional details concerning the development of other endocrine organs, refer to the subsequent Embryology Summaries on the Lymphatic, Digestive, Urinary, and Reproductive systems.

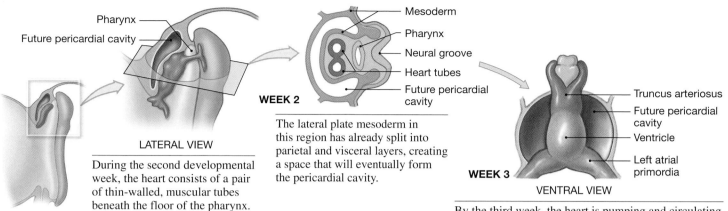

WEEK 2

LATERAL VIEW

During the second developmental week, the heart consists of a pair of thin-walled, muscular tubes beneath the floor of the pharynx.

The lateral plate mesoderm in this region has already split into parietal and visceral layers, creating a space that will eventually form the pericardial cavity.

WEEK 3

VENTRAL VIEW

By the third week, the heart is pumping and circulating blood. The cardiac tubes have fused, producing a heart with a single central chamber. Two large veins bring blood to the heart, and a single large artery, the **truncus arteriosus**, carries blood to the general circulation.

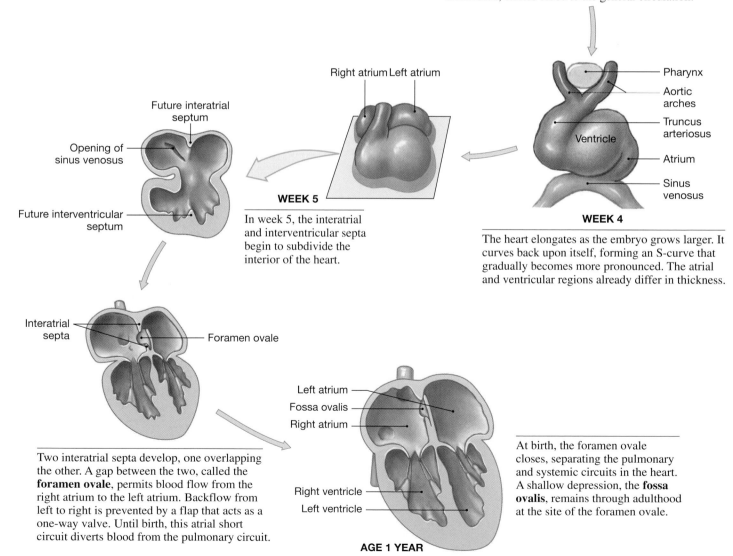

WEEK 5

In week 5, the interatrial and interventricular septa begin to subdivide the interior of the heart.

WEEK 4

The heart elongates as the embryo grows larger. It curves back upon itself, forming an S-curve that gradually becomes more pronounced. The atrial and ventricular regions already differ in thickness.

Two interatrial septa develop, one overlapping the other. A gap between the two, called the **foramen ovale**, permits blood flow from the right atrium to the left atrium. Backflow from left to right is prevented by a flap that acts as a one-way valve. Until birth, this atrial short circuit diverts blood from the pulmonary circuit.

AGE 1 YEAR

At birth, the foramen ovale closes, separating the pulmonary and systemic circuits in the heart. A shallow depression, the **fossa ovalis**, remains through adulthood at the site of the foramen ovale.

EMBRYOLOGY SUMMARY 15: THE DEVELOPMENT OF THE HEART

THE AORTIC ARCHES

An **aortic arch** carries arterial blood through each of the *pharyngeal arches*. In the dorsal pharyngeal wall, these vessels fuse to create the **dorsal aorta**, which distributes blood throughout the body. The arches are usually numbered from I to VI, corresponding to the pharyngeal arches.

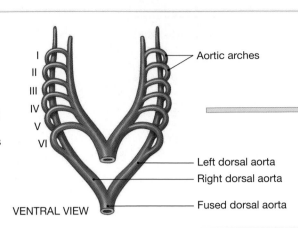

I
II
III
IV
V
VI

Aortic arches

Left dorsal aorta
Right dorsal aorta
Fused dorsal aorta

VENTRAL VIEW

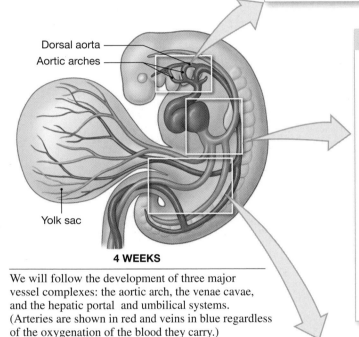

Dorsal aorta
Aortic arches

Yolk sac

4 WEEKS

We will follow the development of three major vessel complexes: the aortic arch, the venae cavae, and the hepatic portal and umbilical systems. (Arteries are shown in red and veins in blue regardless of the oxygenation of the blood they carry.)

THE VENAE CAVAE

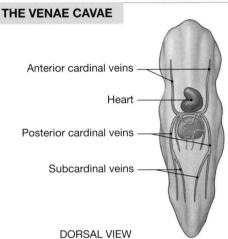

Anterior cardinal veins

Heart

Posterior cardinal veins

Subcardinal veins

DORSAL VIEW

The early venous circulation draining the tissues of the body wall, limbs, and head centers around the paired **anterior cardinal veins**, **posterior cardinal veins**, and **subcardinal veins**.

THE HEPATIC PORTAL AND UMBILICAL VESSELS

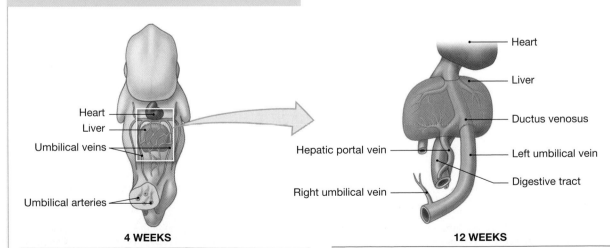

Heart
Liver
Umbilical veins

Umbilical arteries

4 WEEKS

Paired **umbilical arteries** deliver blood to the placenta. At 4 weeks, paired **umbilical veins** return blood to capillary networks in the liver. Veins running along the length of the digestive tract have extensive interconnections.

Heart

Liver

Ductus venosus

Hepatic portal vein

Left umbilical vein

Right umbilical vein

Digestive tract

12 WEEKS

By week 12, the right umbilical vein disintegrates, and the blood from the placenta travels along a single umbilical vein. The **ductus venosus** allows some venous blood to bypass the liver. The veins draining the digestive tract have fused, forming the hepatic portal vein.

EMBRYOLOGY SUMMARY 16: THE DEVELOPMENT OF THE CARDIOVASCULAR SYSTEM

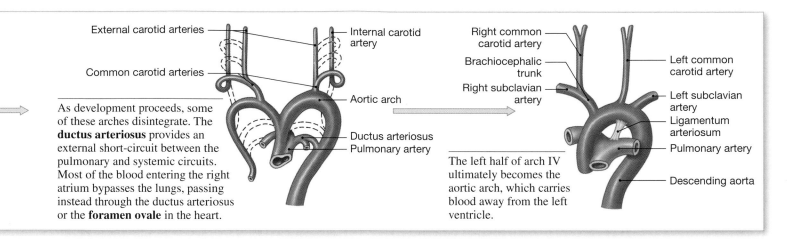

As development proceeds, some of these arches disintegrate. The **ductus arteriosus** provides an external short-circuit between the pulmonary and systemic circuits. Most of the blood entering the right atrium bypasses the lungs, passing instead through the ductus arteriosus or the **foramen ovale** in the heart.

The left half of arch IV ultimately becomes the aortic arch, which carries blood away from the left ventricle.

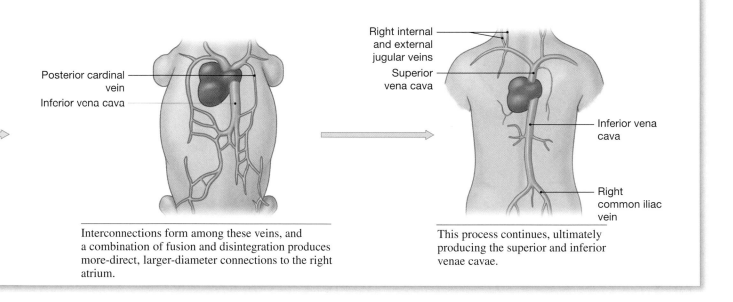

Interconnections form among these veins, and a combination of fusion and disintegration produces more-direct, larger-diameter connections to the right atrium.

This process continues, ultimately producing the superior and inferior venae cavae.

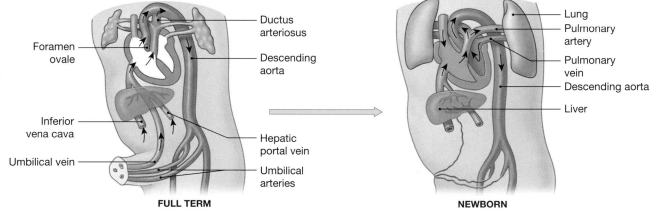

FULL TERM

Shortly before birth, blood returning from the placenta travels through the liver in the ductus venosus to reach the inferior vena cava. Much of the blood delivered by the venae cavae bypasses the lungs by traveling through the foramen ovale and the ductus arteriosus.

NEWBORN

At birth, pressures drop in the pleural cavities as the chest expands and the infant takes its first breath. The pulmonary vessels dilate, and blood flow to the lungs increases. Pressure falls in the right atrium, and the higher left atrial pressures close the valve that guards the foramen ovale. Smooth muscles contract the ductus arteriosus, which ultimately converts to the **ligamentum arteriosum**, a fibrous strand.

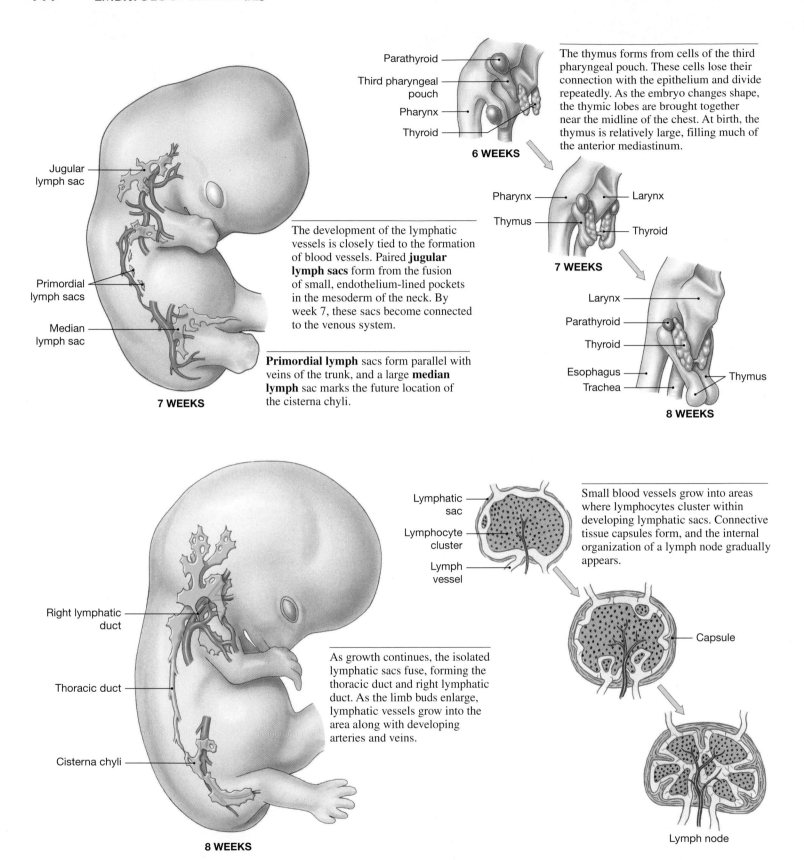

Parathyroid

Third pharyngeal pouch

Pharynx

Thyroid

6 WEEKS

The thymus forms from cells of the third pharyngeal pouch. These cells lose their connection with the epithelium and divide repeatedly. As the embryo changes shape, the thymic lobes are brought together near the midline of the chest. At birth, the thymus is relatively large, filling much of the anterior mediastinum.

Pharynx

Thymus

Larynx

Thyroid

7 WEEKS

Larynx

Parathyroid

Thyroid

Esophagus

Trachea

Thymus

8 WEEKS

Jugular lymph sac

Primordial lymph sacs

Median lymph sac

7 WEEKS

The development of the lymphatic vessels is closely tied to the formation of blood vessels. Paired **jugular lymph sacs** form from the fusion of small, endothelium-lined pockets in the mesoderm of the neck. By week 7, these sacs become connected to the venous system.

Primordial lymph sacs form parallel with veins of the trunk, and a large **median lymph** sac marks the future location of the cisterna chyli.

Right lymphatic duct

Thoracic duct

Cisterna chyli

8 WEEKS

As growth continues, the isolated lymphatic sacs fuse, forming the thoracic duct and right lymphatic duct. As the limb buds enlarge, lymphatic vessels grow into the area along with developing arteries and veins.

Lymphatic sac

Lymphocyte cluster

Lymph vessel

Small blood vessels grow into areas where lymphocytes cluster within developing lymphatic sacs. Connective tissue capsules form, and the internal organization of a lymph node gradually appears.

Capsule

Lymph node

EMBRYOLOGY SUMMARY 17: THE DEVELOPMENT OF THE LYMPHATIC SYSTEM

THE LUNGS

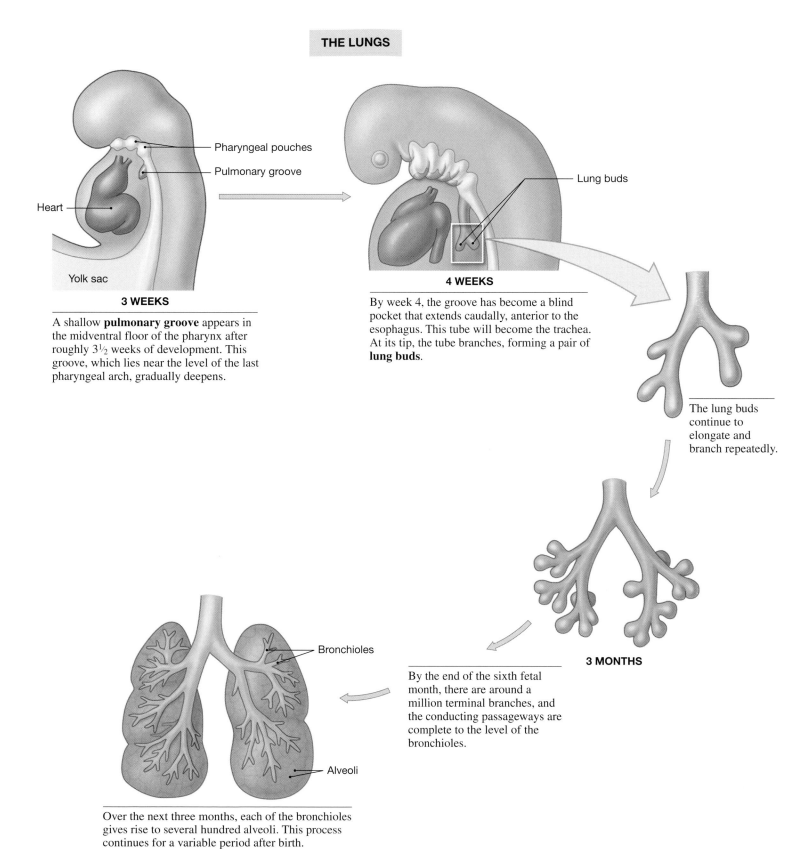

Pharyngeal pouches

Pulmonary groove

Heart

Yolk sac

3 WEEKS

A shallow **pulmonary groove** appears in the midventral floor of the pharynx after roughly 3½ weeks of development. This groove, which lies near the level of the last pharyngeal arch, gradually deepens.

4 WEEKS

Lung buds

By week 4, the groove has become a blind pocket that extends caudally, anterior to the esophagus. This tube will become the trachea. At its tip, the tube branches, forming a pair of **lung buds**.

The lung buds continue to elongate and branch repeatedly.

3 MONTHS

By the end of the sixth fetal month, there are around a million terminal branches, and the conducting passageways are complete to the level of the bronchioles.

Bronchioles

Alveoli

Over the next three months, each of the bronchioles gives rise to several hundred alveoli. This process continues for a variable period after birth.

EMBRYOLOGY SUMMARY **18**: THE DEVELOPMENT OF THE RESPIRATORY SYSTEM—*PART I*

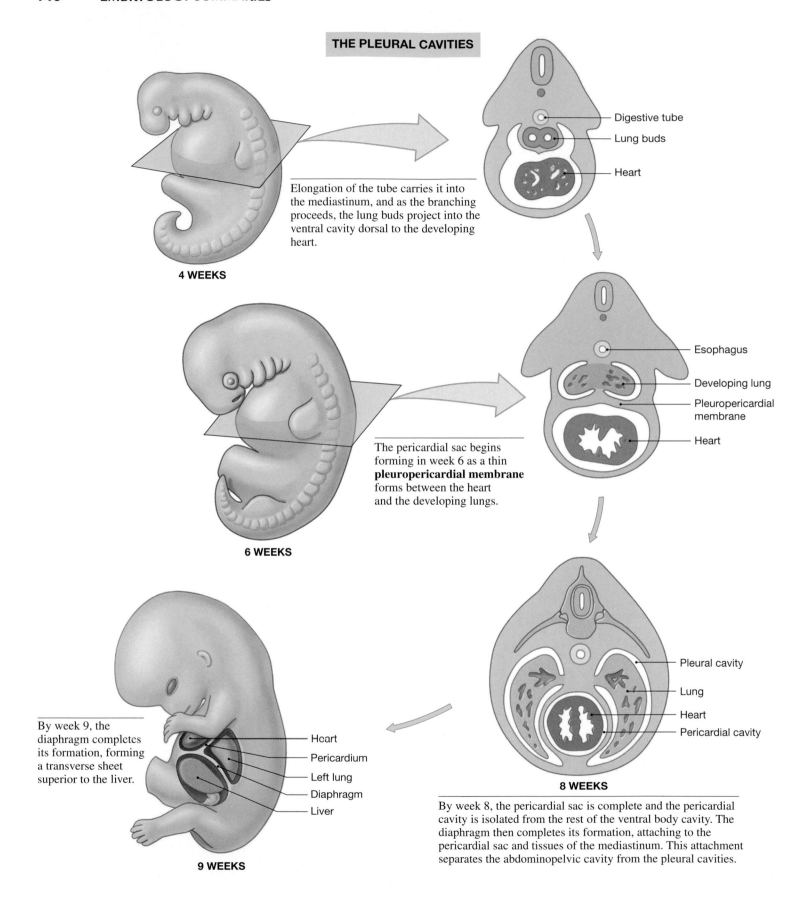

THE PLEURAL CAVITIES

Elongation of the tube carries it into the mediastinum, and as the branching proceeds, the lung buds project into the ventral cavity dorsal to the developing heart.

4 WEEKS

- Digestive tube
- Lung buds
- Heart

The pericardial sac begins forming in week 6 as a thin **pleuropericardial membrane** forms between the heart and the developing lungs.

6 WEEKS

- Esophagus
- Developing lung
- Pleuropericardial membrane
- Heart

By week 9, the diaphragm completes its formation, forming a transverse sheet superior to the liver.

- Heart
- Pericardium
- Left lung
- Diaphragm
- Liver

9 WEEKS

- Pleural cavity
- Lung
- Heart
- Pericardial cavity

8 WEEKS

By week 8, the pericardial sac is complete and the pericardial cavity is isolated from the rest of the ventral body cavity. The diaphragm then completes its formation, attaching to the pericardial sac and tissues of the mediastinum. This attachment separates the abdominopelvic cavity from the pleural cavities.

EMBRYOLOGY SUMMARY 18: THE DEVELOPMENT OF THE RESPIRATORY SYSTEM—PART II

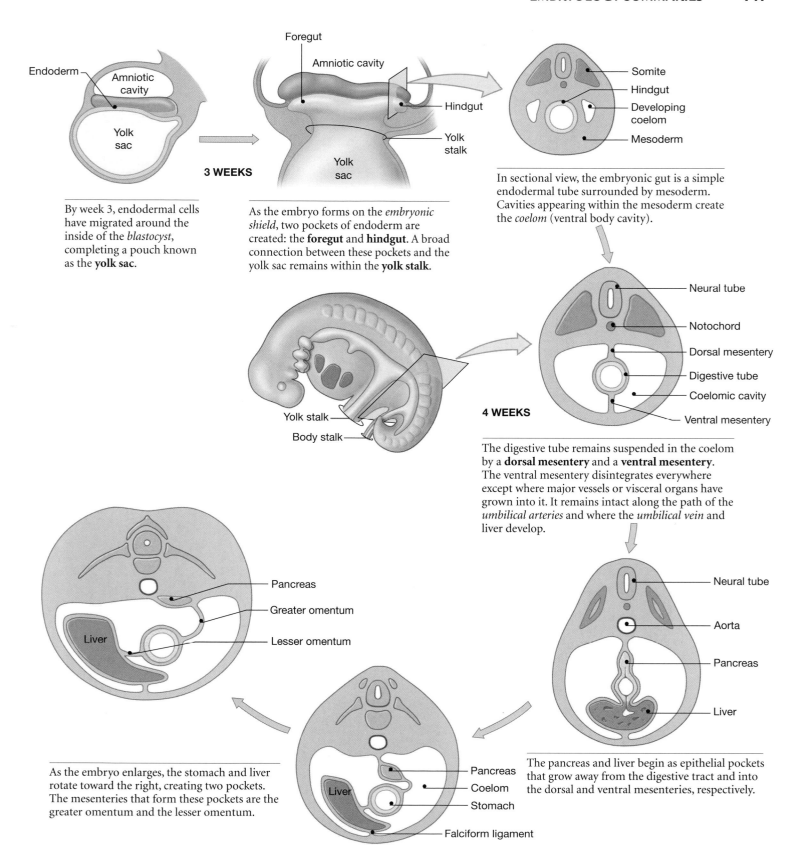

By week 3, endodermal cells have migrated around the inside of the *blastocyst*, completing a pouch known as the **yolk sac**.

3 WEEKS

As the embryo forms on the *embryonic shield*, two pockets of endoderm are created: the **foregut** and **hindgut**. A broad connection between these pockets and the yolk sac remains within the **yolk stalk**.

In sectional view, the embryonic gut is a simple endodermal tube surrounded by mesoderm. Cavities appearing within the mesoderm create the *coelom* (ventral body cavity).

4 WEEKS

The digestive tube remains suspended in the coelom by a **dorsal mesentery** and a **ventral mesentery**. The ventral mesentery disintegrates everywhere except where major vessels or visceral organs have grown into it. It remains intact along the path of the *umbilical arteries* and where the *umbilical vein* and liver develop.

The pancreas and liver begin as epithelial pockets that grow away from the digestive tract and into the dorsal and ventral mesenteries, respectively.

As the embryo enlarges, the stomach and liver rotate toward the right, creating two pockets. The mesenteries that form these pockets are the greater omentum and the lesser omentum.

EMBRYOLOGY SUMMARY 19: THE DEVELOPMENT OF THE DIGESTIVE SYSTEM—*PART I*

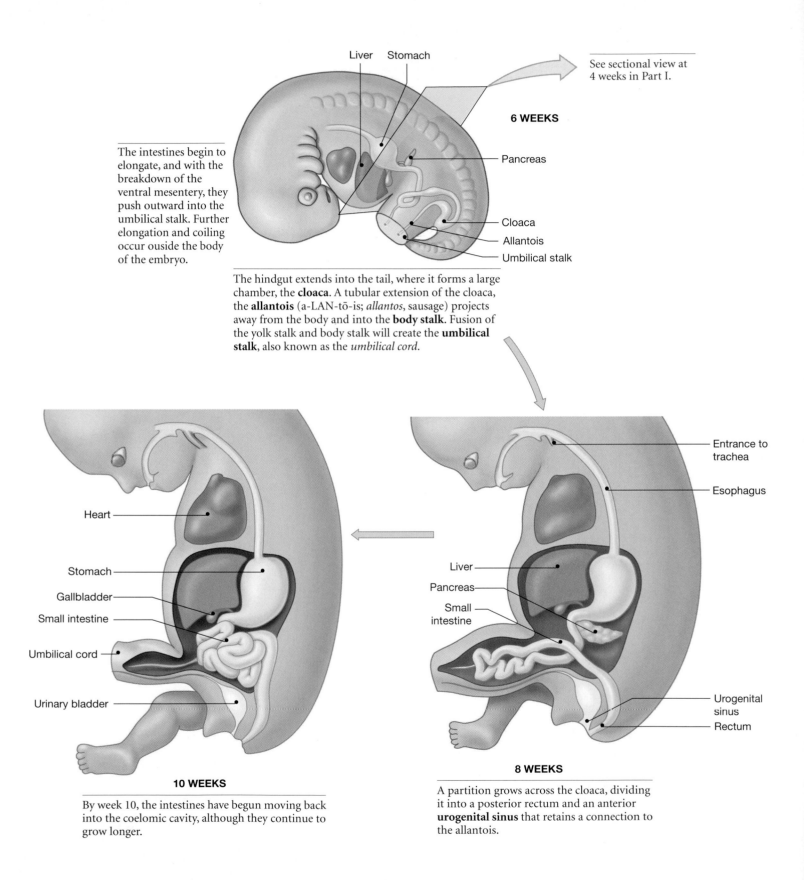

Liver   Stomach

See sectional view at 4 weeks in Part I.

6 WEEKS

The intestines begin to elongate, and with the breakdown of the ventral mesentery, they push outward into the umbilical stalk. Further elongation and coiling occur ouside the body of the embryo.

Pancreas

Cloaca

Allantois

Umbilical stalk

The hindgut extends into the tail, where it forms a large chamber, the **cloaca**. A tubular extension of the cloaca, the **allantois** (a-LAN-tō-is; *allantos*, sausage) projects away from the body and into the **body stalk**. Fusion of the yolk stalk and body stalk will create the **umbilical stalk**, also known as the *umbilical cord*.

Heart

Stomach

Gallbladder

Small intestine

Umbilical cord

Urinary bladder

10 WEEKS

By week 10, the intestines have begun moving back into the coelomic cavity, although they continue to grow longer.

Entrance to trachea

Esophagus

Liver

Pancreas

Small intestine

Urogenital sinus

Rectum

8 WEEKS

A partition grows across the cloaca, dividing it into a posterior rectum and an anterior **urogenital sinus** that retains a connection to the allantois.

EMBRYOLOGY SUMMARY **19**: THE DEVELOPMENT OF THE DIGESTIVE SYSTEM—*PART II*

The kidneys develop in stages along the axis of the **urogenital ridge**, a thickened area beneath the dorso-lateral wall of the coelomic cavity.

Kidney development proceeds along the cranial/caudal axis of this ridge, beginning with the formation of the **pronephros**, continuing along the **mesonephros**, and ending with the development of the **metanephros**.

The pronephros consists of a series of tubules (generally 7 pairs) that appears within the **nephrotome**, the narrow band of mesoderm between the somites and the lateral plate.

The pronephric tubules are very small and nonfunctional, and they disintegrate almost at once. The only significant contribution of the pronephros is the formation of a pair of **pronephric ducts** that grow caudally until they connect to the *cloaca*.

3½ WEEKS

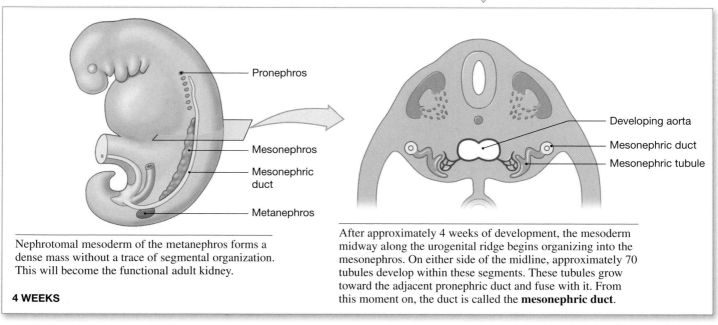

Nephrotomal mesoderm of the metanephros forms a dense mass without a trace of segmental organization. This will become the functional adult kidney.

4 WEEKS

After approximately 4 weeks of development, the mesoderm midway along the urogenital ridge begins organizing into the mesonephros. On either side of the midline, approximately 70 tubules develop within these segments. These tubules grow toward the adjacent pronephric duct and fuse with it. From this moment on, the duct is called the **mesonephric duct**.

EMBRYOLOGY SUMMARY 20: THE DEVELOPMENT OF THE URINARY SYSTEM—*PART I*

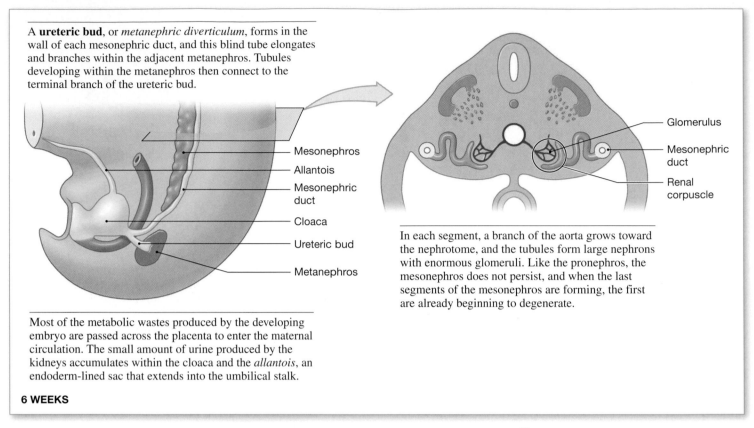

A **ureteric bud**, or *metanephric diverticulum*, forms in the wall of each mesonephric duct, and this blind tube elongates and branches within the adjacent metanephros. Tubules developing within the metanephros then connect to the terminal branch of the ureteric bud.

Mesonephros
Allantois
Mesonephric duct
Cloaca
Ureteric bud
Metanephros

Glomerulus
Mesonephric duct
Renal corpuscle

In each segment, a branch of the aorta grows toward the nephrotome, and the tubules form large nephrons with enormous glomeruli. Like the pronephros, the mesonephros does not persist, and when the last segments of the mesonephros are forming, the first are already beginning to degenerate.

Most of the metabolic wastes produced by the developing embryo are passed across the placenta to enter the maternal circulation. The small amount of urine produced by the kidneys accumulates within the cloaca and the *allantois*, an endoderm-lined sac that extends into the umbilical stalk.

6 WEEKS

Nephron
Collecting tubule
Collecting duct

Mesonephric duct
Degenerating mesonephros

Developing metanephros

Collecting system

Major calyx

Urinary bladder
Urogenital sinus
Rectum

Metanephros

Ureter

Ureteric bud

12 WEEKS

The kidneys begin producing filtrate by the third developmental month. The filtrate does not contain waste products, as they are excreted at the placenta for removal and elimination by the maternal kidneys. The sterile filtrate mixes with the amniotic fluid and is swallowed by the fetus and reabsorbed across the lining of the digestive tract.

The ureteric bud branches within the metanephros, creating the calyces and the collecting system. The nephrons, which form within the mesoderm of the metanephros, tap into the collecting tubules.

8 WEEKS

Near the end of the second developmental month, the cloaca is subdivided into a dorsal rectum and a ventral **urogenital sinus**. The proximal portions of the allantois persist as the **urinary bladder**, and the connection between the bladder and an opening on the body surface will form the **urethra**.

EMBRYOLOGY SUMMARY 20: THE DEVELOPMENT OF THE URINARY SYSTEM—*PART II*

SEXUALLY INDIFFERENT STAGES
(WEEKS 3–6)

DEVELOPMENT OF THE GONADS

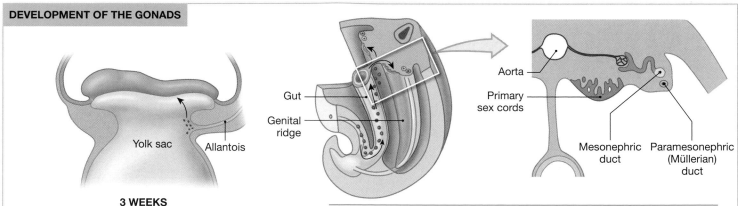

3 WEEKS

During the third week, endodermal cells migrate from the wall of the yolk sac near the allantois to the dorsal wall of the abdominal cavity. These primordial germ cells enter the **genital ridges** that parallel the mesonephros.

Each ridge has a thick epithelium continuous with columns of cells, the **primary sex cords**, that extend into the center (medulla) of the ridge. Anterior to each mesonephric duct, a duct forms that has no connection to the kidneys. This is the **paramesonephric** (*Müllerian*) **duct**; it extends along the genital ridge and continues toward the cloaca. At this sexually indifferent stage, male embryos cannot be distinguished from female embryos.

DEVELOPMENT OF DUCTS AND ACCESSORY ORGANS

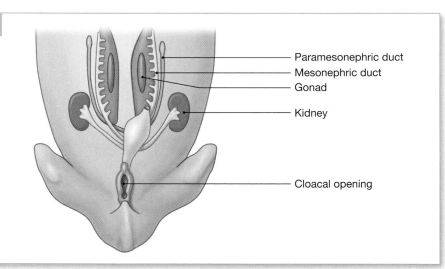

Both sexes have mesonephric and paramesonephric ducts at this stage. Unless exposed to androgens, the embryo—regardless of its genetic sex—will develop into a female. In a normal male embryo, cells in the core (medulla) of the genital ridge begin producing testosterone sometime after week 6. Testosterone triggers the changes in the duct system and external genitalia that are detailed on the following page.

DEVELOPMENT OF EXTERNAL GENITALIA

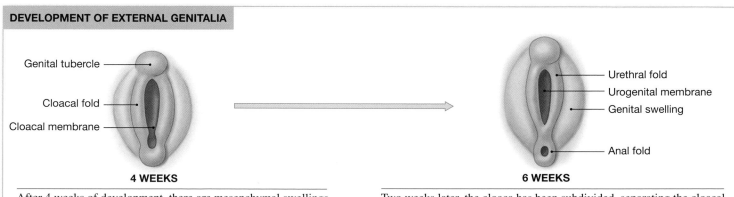

4 WEEKS

After 4 weeks of development, there are mesenchymal swellings called **cloacal folds** around the **cloacal membrane** (the cloaca does not open to the exterior). The **genital tubercle** forms the glans of the penis in males and the clitoris in females.

6 WEEKS

Two weeks later, the cloaca has been subdivided, separating the cloacal membrane into a posterior *anal membrane*, bounded by the *anal folds*, and an anterior **urogenital membrane**, bounded by the **urethral folds**. A prominent **genital swelling** forms lateral to each urethral fold.

DEVELOPMENT OF THE MALE REPRODUCTIVE SYSTEM

DEVELOPMENT OF THE TESTES

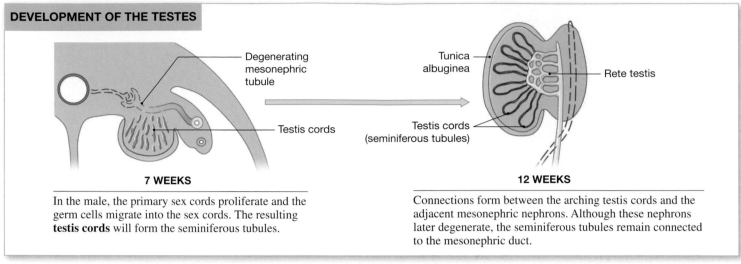

7 WEEKS

In the male, the primary sex cords proliferate and the germ cells migrate into the sex cords. The resulting **testis cords** will form the seminiferous tubules.

12 WEEKS

Connections form between the arching testis cords and the adjacent mesonephric nephrons. Although these nephrons later degenerate, the seminiferous tubules remain connected to the mesonephric duct.

DEVELOPMENT OF MALE DUCTS AND ACCESSORY ORGANS

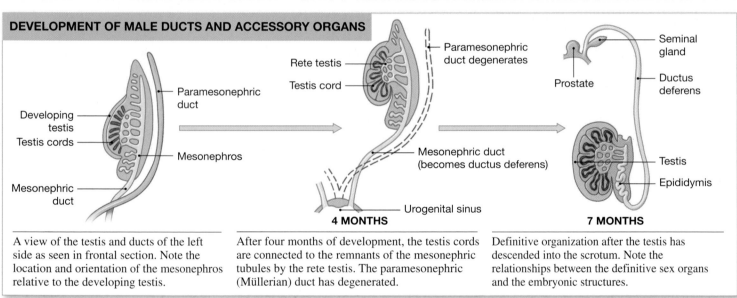

4 MONTHS

7 MONTHS

A view of the testis and ducts of the left side as seen in frontal section. Note the location and orientation of the mesonephros relative to the developing testis.

After four months of development, the testis cords are connected to the remnants of the mesonephric tubules by the rete testis. The paramesonephric (Müllerian) duct has degenerated.

Definitive organization after the testis has descended into the scrotum. Note the relationships between the definitive sex organs and the embryonic structures.

DEVELOPMENT OF MALE EXTERNAL GENITALIA

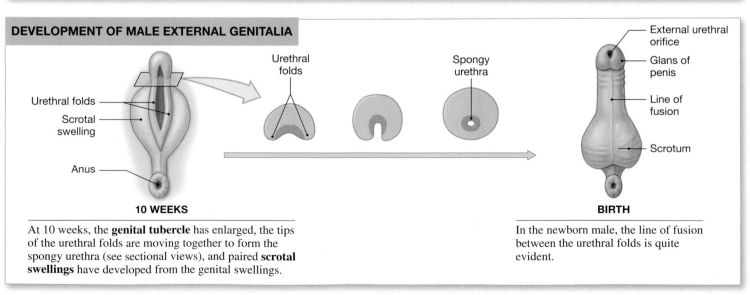

10 WEEKS

At 10 weeks, the **genital tubercle** has enlarged, the tips of the urethral folds are moving together to form the spongy urethra (see sectional views), and paired **scrotal swellings** have developed from the genital swellings.

BIRTH

In the newborn male, the line of fusion between the urethral folds is quite evident.

DEVELOPMENT OF THE FEMALE REPRODUCTIVE SYSTEM

DEVELOPMENT OF THE OVARIES

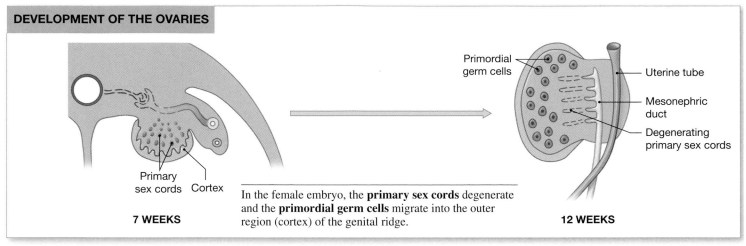

Primordial germ cells

Uterine tube

Mesonephric duct

Degenerating primary sex cords

Primary sex cords   Cortex

In the female embryo, the **primary sex cords** degenerate and the **primordial germ cells** migrate into the outer region (cortex) of the genital ridge.

7 WEEKS

12 WEEKS

DEVELOPMENT OF FEMALE DUCTS AND ACCESSORY ORGANS

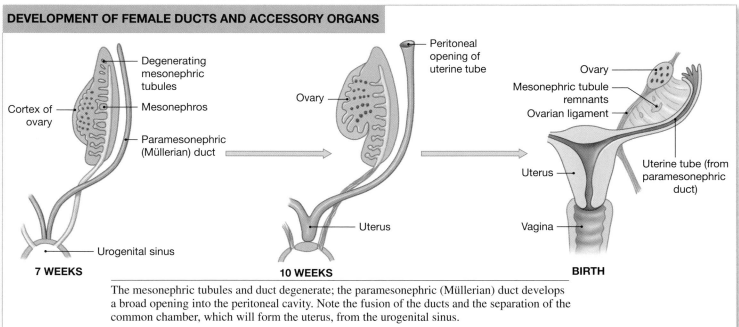

Degenerating mesonephric tubules

Mesonephros

Cortex of ovary

Paramesonephric (Müllerian) duct

Urogenital sinus

Peritoneal opening of uterine tube

Ovary

Uterus

Ovary

Mesonephric tubule remnants

Ovarian ligament

Uterus

Uterine tube (from paramesonephric duct)

Vagina

7 WEEKS

10 WEEKS

BIRTH

The mesonephric tubules and duct degenerate; the paramesonephric (Müllerian) duct develops a broad opening into the peritoneal cavity. Note the fusion of the ducts and the separation of the common chamber, which will form the uterus, from the urogenital sinus.

COMPARISON OF MALE AND FEMALE EXTERNAL GENITALIA

Males	Females
Penis	Clitoris
Corpora cavernosa	Erectile tissue
Corpus spongiosum	Vestibular bulbs
Proximal shaft of penis	Labia minora
Spongy urethra	Vestibule
Bulbourethral glands	Greater vestibular glands
Scrotum	Labia majora

DEVELOPMENT OF FEMALE EXTERNAL GENITALIA

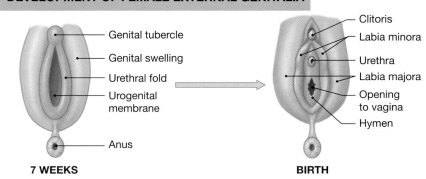

Genital tubercle

Genital swelling

Urethral fold

Urogenital membrane

Anus

Clitoris

Labia minora

Urethra

Labia majora

Opening to vagina

Hymen

7 WEEKS

BIRTH

In the female, the urethral folds do not fuse; they develop into the labia minora. The genital swellings will form the labia majora. The genital tubercle develops into the clitoris. The urethra opens to the exterior immediately posterior to the clitoris. The hymen remains as an elaboration of the urogenital membrane.

EMBRYOLOGY SUMMARY **21:** THE DEVELOPMENT OF THE REPRODUCTIVE SYSTEM—*PART III*